H. Ishihara, A.H. Giesecke

Fluid Volume Monitoring with Glucose Dilution

H. Ishihara, A.H. Giesecke

Fluid Volume Monitoring with Glucose Dilution

With 55 Figures

Springer

Hironori Ishihara, M.D.
Associate Professor, Department of Anesthesiology
University of Hirosaki School of Medicine
5 Zaifu-cho, Hirosaki 036-8562, Japan

Adolph H. Giesecke, M.D.
Emeritus Professor, former Jenkins Professor and Chairman
Anesthesiology and Pain Management
University of Texas Southwestern Medical Center
5323 Harry Hines Blvd., Dallas, Texas 75390-9068, U.S.A.

ISBN-10 4-431-47192-8 Springer Tokyo Berlin Heidelberg New York
ISBN-13 978-4-431-47192-9 Springer Tokyo Berlin Heidelberg New York

Library of Congress Control Number: 2006936621

Springer is a part of Springer Science+Business Media
springer.com

Printed in Japan

Typesetting: SNP Best-set Typesetter Ltd., Hong Kong
Printing and binding: Shinano Inc., Japan

Printed on acid-free paper

Foreword

Academic medicine can be very satisfying. I am pleased when I see one of my residents takes excellent care of a seriously injured patient. I am pleased when a junior member of the faculty publishes a really good paper. I am pleased when the program attracts an especially good group of residents. Sources of satisfaction can be multiple when one is a teacher, but Ishihara has presented me with one of the best.

He has taken an idea, which arose from a related research project in 1979, and devoted his career to exploring every ramification and answering almost every question related to it. The related research had to do with the mechanism of hyperglycemia in various states of general and regional anesthesia. The idea that triggered his imagination was to use glucose as a marker for the measurement of central extracellular fluid (ECF) volume. His exhaustive work forms the material for this book.

He has studied animals and humans, healthy people and sick. He has answered the pressing questions, whether simple or complex. He has compared his technique to the recognized gold standards of analysis in a wide variety of complex clinical situations. When I say a wide variety of complex clinical situations, I mean patients in his intensive care unit with severe hemorrhagic hypovolemia, congestive heart failure, respiratory failure on long-term ventilator support, adrenal insufficiency, and metabolic imbalance on insulin infusions. His studies have always been directed to the goal of improved decision making in the area of fluid therapy and inotropic support. His dedication has paid off. He has the answers. The initial distribution volume of glucose (IDVG) is a valuable marker of central ECF volume and a valuable guide to therapy. Why then has it not become more popular? I believe because it is too simple and does not generate profit for anybody but the patient. It does not involve computers or expensive new drugs. It does not posses an army of salesmen who promote its virtues in the coffee rooms of relaxing anesthesiologists and intensivists.

His work is detailed, exhaustive, critically analyzed, and correct. I hope that the world recognizes it and makes better use of this valuable tool.

Adolph H. Giesecke, M.D.
Emeritus Professor, former Jenkins Professor and Chairman
Anesthesiology and Pain Management
University of Texas Southwestern Medical Center
Dallas, TX 75390-9068, U.S.A.
Adolph.giesecke@utsouthwestern.edu

Introduction

A clinically important misinterpretation of cardiac preload or circulating blood volume could cause serious consequences in critically ill patients. However, many physicians do not possess a proper knowledge of fluid volume assessment. They are generally not interested in fluid volume assessment, but rather are interested in the underlying pathology and/or cardiac function of their patients. Accordingly, decision making about fluid volume loading, fluid restriction, or administration of vasoactive drugs may vary among physicians, depending solely on their clinical experience in the absence of evidence-based measurement, leading to a significant increase in morbidity as well as length of hospital stay in the critically ill.

When I started anesthesia, almost 30 years ago, surgeons sometimes complained about our fluid management, saying, 'You gave too much fluid to my patient. We have to give blood and diuretics to remove excess fluid in our surgical ward.' In contrast, 'You gave insufficient amounts of fluid to my patient. We have to give volume loading in our surgical ward.' However, we could not adequately respond to the surgeon's criticism, because at that time we had no clinically relevant marker to assess fluid volume status in the body. Thus, I became interested in fluid management and began to seek a clinically relevant evaluation of fluid volume status. In 1979, fortunately, I had a chance to work as a visiting research fellow in the Department of Anesthesiology, University of Texas at Dallas, where the 'Parkland formula,' using a large amount of crystalloid solution, is famous worldwide. I met Professor Adolph Giesecke, who was an expert in this field in anesthesiology. He gave me a research project of intravenous glucose challenge testing during various types of anesthesia, including spinal anesthesia, in dogs. Based on this study, I was able to understand the relationship between glucose clearance and insulin response. During the preparation of the manuscript, we discussed the distribution volume of glucose to interpret the results of our data within 60 min after glucose challenge, but we gave up calculating it because we believed that glucose metabolism would obviously affect the pharmacokinetic behavior of administered glucose.

After I came back to our department in Hirosaki, I found that the magnitude of transient hyperglycemia after a small amount of glucose challenge does not consistently follow acute insulin response in which blood sampling was extended only to 10 min after the challenge. I calculated the distribution volume of glucose, that is, glucose space, with a one-compartment model and found that glucose space decreased during surgery, and that it further decreased when a ganglion-blocking agent was infused during surgery. At that time I did not realize the glucose space was a marker of fluid volume status, but only realized that its reduction may play a role in hyperglycemia observed in the perioperative period. Further detailed description of our early studies is available in the second chapter.

When I started to work in the intensive care unit (ICU) in 1983, the issues regarding assessment of fluid volume status still remained unsolved, yet I remained interested in this field. One day I had a chance to measure glucose space and cardiac output in a girl with pheochromocytoma before and after surgical removal of the tumor. Before measurement, I speculated that obvious changes in plasma catecholamine levels in this patient may affect both glucose metabolism and cardiac output. I found a linear correlation between glucose space and cardiac output in this patient, implying glucose space has potential as a marker of fluid volume status without modification of glucose metabolism. From that point, my colleague and I began to study glucose space as a marker of fluid volume status closely related to cardiac output. In the meantime, I changed the name 'glucose space' to 'initial distribution volume of glucose (IDVG)' because our 'glucose space' does not cover the entire distribution volume of glucose but indicates the distribution volume of the early phase only. Finally, we reached the conclusion that IDVG reflects cardiac preload, even though administered glucose cannot stay in the intravascular compartment, and IDVG is not consistently equivalent as a marker of cardiac preload but rather is more closely related to cardiac output than intrathoracic blood volume.

Measurement of IDVG, however, remains an underutilized, poorly understood technique, even after we published several papers regarding IDVG as a clinically relevant marker of fluid volume. We believe that measurement of IDVG should be more popular because it is simple, quick, safe, reliable, and inexpensive. It can be done in any ICU or operating room where a conventional blood glucose analyzer is readily available, unless patients have excessive hyperglycemia. Although this technique is very simple, the reader should understand its basic concept and the proper measurement technique; otherwise, it may be harmful to the patient. In this volume, I intend to cover all aspects of IDVG measurement including the basic concept, relationship with other fluid volumes, and clinical application of this technique in the ICU, based both on our studies and our experience of more than 4000 IDVG determinations.

I hope that readers are encouraged to routinely use IDVG measurement in a wide range of critical conditions. It is also my sincere wish that some readers will be stimulated to extend the knowledge of subject matter in which deficiencies currently exist.

Hironori Ishihara, M.D.
Associate Professor
Department of Anesthesiology
University of Hirosaki School of Medicine
Hirosaki 036-8562, Japan
ishihara@cc.hirosaki-u.ac.jp

Acknowledgment

I am greatly indebted, first, to Emeritus Professor Akitomo Matsuki, who initially planned to publish this monograph and always encouraged me to write it. He also read and commented on the entire text. Without his enthusiasm, this book would not have been published.

I also wish to express my deepest appreciation to my professional colleagues in the Department of Anesthesiology, University of Hirosaki School of Medicine, particularly to Professor Kazuyoshi Hirota, as well as to other persons outside the Department for their continued support and understanding of the study: Emeritus Professor John W.R. McIntyre (Edmonton, Canada) who taught me how to write scientific papers in the 1990s, Professor Bernhard Panning (Hannover, Germany), and Professor and Chairman Dominique Grimaud (Nice, France), who sent Dr. Oliver Rose and Dr. Jean Christophe Orban to me to do collaboration studies in this field.

I am particularly grateful to Emeritus Professor Adolph H. Giesecke, who not only read and edited the entire text as a coauthor but also contributed a generous foreword. And finally, I thank Mrs. Koh Mikami for her excellent secretarial services, and the staffs of Springer Japan for continued editorial and production excellence.

Hironori Ishihara

Contents

1. Principle of Dilution Volumetry

Dilution Volumetry and Pharmacokinetic Models

Methods for measuring blood volume or extracellular fluid volume in humans are based on dilution volumetry utilizing an aliquot of an indicator substance (Table 1-1).

Dilution volumetry is based on the principle of conservation of mass, which means that the total mass of a substance after dispersion in the fluid compartment will be the same as the total injected into the compartment. The distribution volume of the indicator can be calculated simply by the following formula:

Distribution volume = dose/concentration

where dose is the amount of a given indicator and concentration is the concentration of an indicator in the compartment when mixed completely in the compartment before its elimination. As most nonisotopic indicators have a short half-life, the indicators begin to be cleared from the compartment immediately after injection. Thus, a one-compartment or a more-complicated model is generally applied to determine the distribution volume of such indicators (Fig. 1-1). In the one-compartment model, the volume of distribution (V_d) and plasma concentration at any time t (C) are calculated as follows:

$$V_d = \text{dose}/C_0$$

$$C = (\text{dose}/C_0)\ e^{-kt}$$

where dose = amount of indicator administered, C_0 = initial plasma concentration at time (0) after instantaneous distribution but before the start of elimination, and k = disappearance rate from plasma.

TABLE 1-1. Measurement of body fluid volumes

Volume	Indicators
Total body water	^3H_2O, ^2H_2O, antipyrine, ethanol
Extracellular fluid	^{22}Na, ^{125}I-iothalamate, thiosulfate, inulin, sucrose
Plasma	^{125}I-albumin, Evans blue, indocyanine green, hydroxyethyl starch
Red cell	^{51}Cr, ^{99m}Tc, carbon monoxide, fluorescein

Source: modified from Guyton and Hall (2000b) p 268, table 25-3 with permission from Elsevier

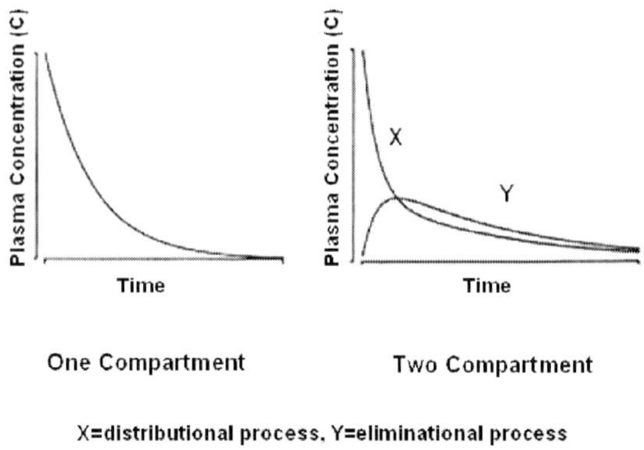

FIG. 1-1. Changes in plasma drug concentration in the one- and two-compartment models. *X*, distributional process; *Y*, elimination process

In the two-compartment model, two distinct phases characterize the curve: distribution and elimination phases. Plasma concentration at any time *t* (C) is calculated as follows:

$$C = A\ e^{-\alpha t} + B\ e^{-\beta t}$$

where α and β are rate constants for distribution and elimination phases, and α is generally greater than β. A and B are intercepts at time zero. The distribution phase begins immediately after intravenous injection of the indicator and reflects the distribution of indicator from the central to the peripheral compartment. The elimination phase follows the initial distribution phase and is characterized by a more-gradual decline in the plasma concentration. This gradual decline reflects the elimination of indicator from the central compartment by renal and hepatic clearance mechanisms. In the very early phase, $A\ e^{-\alpha t}$ contributes to the value of C but after three or four time constants of α contributes almost nothing. In the latter phase, where $A\ e^{-\alpha t}$ becomes vanishingly small, the value of C is simply dependent on $B\ e^{-\beta t}$ (Hull 1991). In some circumstances, such as detailed pharmacokinetic analysis of glucose (Cobelli et al. 1990), models of greater complexity provide a better interpretation of the results.

Initial Distribution Volume

The initial distribution volume, or the central compartment of the kinetic description of drug disposition, is that volume in which a drug appears to mix instantaneously before being distributed throughout the remainder of its distribution volume by mixing, flow, and diffusion. One may speculate that the initial volume of distribution for several drugs is composed mainly of the blood volume and the vessel-rich group of tissues and is determined by cardiac output, regional blood flow, and the characteristics of a particular drug (Ghoneim and Pearson 1990). In the two-compartment model, the initial distribution volume (V_{dI}) is calculated as follows (Fig. 1-2):

$$V_{dI} = \text{dose}/(A + B)$$

where A = intercept at time zero of the distribution phase and B = intercept at time zero of elimination phase.

Thus, if line B is apparently lower compared with A, initial distribution volume of the two-compartment model can be substituted by the distribution volume (V_d) of the one-compartment model. In our glucose space study, we have been using a one-compartment model instead of a two-compartment model to analyze pharmacokinetic variables because the former can be easily calculated even at bedside, and line B of plasma glucose decay curve is apparently lower compared with A, even though V_d is not scientifically identical to V_{dI}.

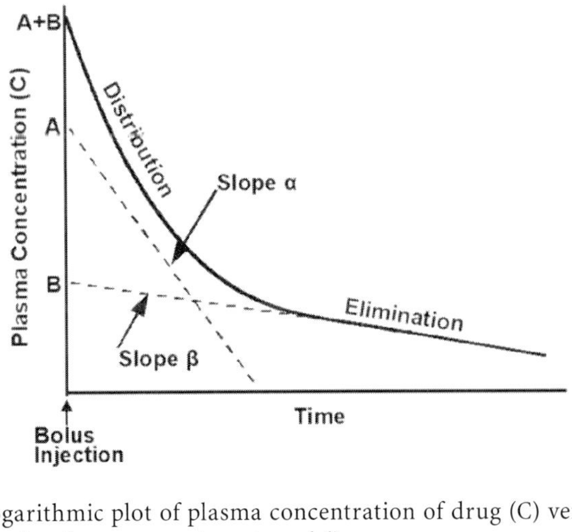

FIG. 1-2. Semilogarithmic plot of plasma concentration of drug (C) versus time after a single bolus injection (two-compartment model)

Accuracies and Controversies in Dilution Volumetry

The principle of dilution volumetry is very simple. However, controversies may exist regarding accuracy in dilution volumetry, such as selection of compartment models and leakage of the indicator substance from the compartment. The latter is discussed in Chapter 8. Dilution volumetry principally requires a steady state of circulation. During data collection, therefore, any changes in circulatory states should be avoided. An infusion rate of glucose for routine fluid management should be continued without a large variability, preferably using an electric fluid pump during the measurement procedure when glucose is used as an indicator for dilution volumetry. Additionally, some technical drawbacks and controversies in interpretation of the measurement exist.

Molecular Weight of Indicators

Distribution volume may change depending on the indicator substance used even if several indicator substances distribute in the same compartments (Jones and Wardrop 2000). Smaller indicator molecules have larger distribution volumes. For example, the distribution volume of ^{125}I-albumin (molecular weight, 69 000) was 5.6% larger than that of ^{125}I-fibrinogen (molecular weight, 330 000) (Tschaikowsky et al. 1997), partly because a significant amount of albumin leaves the intravascular space even during the first 10 min after injection, although the capillary permeability for albumin molecules is 1/1000 that for water molecules (Guyton and Hall 2000a). Consequently, a higher molecular weight is desirable for a plasma volume marker (Tschaikowsky et al. 1997; Thorborg and Haupt 2000). In contrast, the capillary permeability for glucose molecules is 0.6 times that for water molecules, indicating that glucose molecules can rapidly distribute into the extravascular compartment (Table 1-2) (Guyton and Hall 2000a).

Mixing Period

The indicator substance must reach a uniform concentration in the compartment before the sample is taken. Underestimation of circulating blood volume (CBV) may occur when data are calculated before mixing is completed. Although some reports recommended using data at 5 min or thereafter to calculate the distribution volume of indocyanine green (ICG) (Sekimoto et al. 1997; Haller et al. 1993), data collection often began at

TABLE 1-2. Relative permeability of muscular capillary pores to different-sized molecules

Substance	Molecular weight	Permeability
Water	18	1.00
NaCl	58.5	0.96
Urea	60	0.8
Glucose	180	0.6
Sucrose	342	0.4
Inulin	5000	0.2
Myoglobin	17600	0.03
Hemoglobin	68000	0.01
Albumin	69000	0.001

Source: from Guyton and Hall (2000a) p 164, table 16-1 (with permission from Elsevier)

2–3 min postinjection (Haruna et al. 1998), and an underestimation of the plasma volume even in the presence of low cardiac output states would be clinically negligible (Rehm et al. 1998; Henthorn et al. 1989). As judged by the fact that the velocity of water transfer across capillary membranes is about 80 times greater than the linear capillary blood flow, and that the permeability for glucose molecules is 0.6 times that for water molecules, the velocity of glucose transfer across the capillary membrane would be about 50 times greater than the linear capillary blood flow (Guyton and Hall 2000a). Accordingly, a low cardiac output state would yield less underestimation of distribution volume of glucose as compared with indicators for the intravascular volume. In fact, in an obvious low cardiac output state (less than 2.2 l/min m^2), we frequently observed a consistent decline of incremental plasma glucose concentration from the first 1 min postinjection, but a simultaneously administered ICG reached its maximal plasma concentration at 2 min postinjection.

Additionally, there is a finite delay before the first indicator appears at an arterial sampling site following its central venous administration, even though pharmacokinetic analysis has generally been based on the assumption of instantaneous and complete mixing within the sampling site. Mixing transients are known to exist and are expressed as mean transit time (MTT). MTT can be derived from each indicator's dilution curve. MTT is composed of the appearance time, which is the time until the first indicator particle has arrived at the point of detection, and the mean time difference between the occurrence of the first particle and all the following particles (Bindels et al. 2000). In our unpublished observations, when ICG is injected through the central venous line, ICG pulse dye densitometry using a finger probe, which

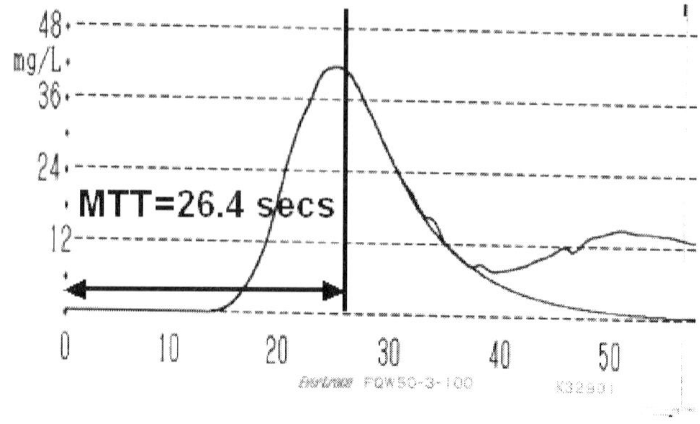

FIG. 1-3. An example of the first circulation curve and prolonged mean transit time (*MTT*) in a patient with acute myocardial infarction recorded at a nostril using indocyanine green (ICG) pulse dye densitometry after injection of ICG through the central vein

is placed closely to a radial artery sampling site, usually showed an MTT of less than 20 s. However, we found MTT of longer than 20 s in some critically ill patients (Fig. 1-3). Therefore, prolonged MTT may also produce underestimation of the distribution volume if the MTT is not taken into account. When MTT of ICG is obviously prolonged, the regression line after MTT should be back-extrapolated to the time point of the MTT for the first circulation curve of ICG.

Duration of Injection

Because the distribution volume of indicators is derived from the formula based on a single bolus intravenous injection, the duration of the injection may affect the result of the calculated distribution volume. The higher disappearance rate from plasma and the longer the duration, the greater the overestimation will be. Using a mathematical equation proposed by Loo and Riegelman (1970), this overestimation can be calculated as follows:

$$\text{Overestimation} = kt/(1 - \exp(-kt))$$

where k is the disappearance rate from plasma (per minute) and t (in minutes) is the duration of injection. When glucose is given over 30 s and the glucose disappearance rate from plasma is 0.07/min, an overestimation of initial distribution volume of glucose (IDVG) calculated by using a one-compartment model will be approximately 1.8% as compared with a single bolus intravenous injection. In our early clinical studies (Ishihara et al. 1993, 1999, 2000c), both 25 ml 20% glucose (5 g) and 10 ml ICG (25 mg) were infused over 30 s instead of as a single bolus injection, as the mixing volume of two indicators in a syringe was 35 ml. Using the foregoing formula, IDVG and ICG-derived plasma volume (PV-ICG) were found to overestimate the value less than 2% for the former and less than 9% for the latter. Thus, a 30-s infusion would have no significant impact clinically on IDVG determination but has a significant impact on PV-ICG determination.

2. Early Studies of Glucose Space

Early Glucose Space Studies

Distribution volume of glucose is also called glucose space. Wick et al. (1950) measured the glucose space of rabbits by dilution volumetry using ^{14}C-labeled glucose. Dilution of the injected glucose was completed in 20 min, and no further dilution took place in 3 h or more. Accordingly, blood samples were collected at 20 min postinjection. Glucose space was close to the thiocyanate space, which is a marker of the extracellular fluid (ECF) volume. Glucose space of eviscerated, nephrectomized, and intact rabbits was 270, 260, and 310 ml/kg, respectively.

Nonlabeled glucose has not generally been used as an indicator for dilution volumetry because the plasma glucose concentration after glucose injection may also be influenced by glucose utilization, endogenous glucose production, urinary loss of glucose, and the continuous infusion of glucose throughout the procedure, as reported by Wick et al. In the 1970s there were a few reports describing glucose space by using nonlabeled glucose (Wilmore et al. 1976; Rosenqvist et al. 1976). Reported nonlabeled glucose space in healthy humans ranges approximately from 150 to 200 ml/kg (Wilmore et al. 1976; Rosensqvist et al. 1976). Wilmore et al. (1976) performed an intravenous glucose tolerance test using rapid injection of 25 g glucose and repeated blood sampling during 3 h postinjection in normal humans, patients burned and with or without sepsis, and burned patients with previous sepsis. The best curve describing the serum glucose decay data points was determined by computer fitting using a one-compartment model (Table 2-1).

Rosenqvist et al. (1976) reported glucose distribution volume in five healthy men with normal body weight after injection of glucose (0.33 g/kg) over 2 min. Blood samples were obtained before injection and then at 5-min intervals for 60 min. Incremental plasma glucose levels above preinjection levels and a one-compartment model were used for calculation of glucose

TABLE 2-1. Glucose space in burned patients with or without sepsis

Patients	Number	Glucose space (ml/kg)	K value (%/min)
Burned patients with sepsis	15	220 ± 15*	2.62 ± 0.47*
Burned patients without sepsis	17	177 ± 10	5.27 ± 0.51
Burned patients with previous sepsis	4	223 ± 10	1.80 ± 0.54
Normal humans	12	152 ± 10	4.01 ± 0.56

Data are shown as mean ± SE
* $P < 0.05$, septic versus burned patients without sepsis
K value, disappearance rate of glucose from plasma
Source: modified from Wilmore et al. (1976), p 721, table 1

TABLE 2-2. Glucose space and K value in five healthy men

Patient	Age (years)	BW (kg)	K value (/min)	Glucose space (ml/kg)
MP	22	69	0.0375 ± 0.0028	146
RF	25	63	0.0249 ± 0.0009	172
PZ	24	83	0.0340 ± 0.0026	177
DW	27	70	0.0202 ± 0.0016	207
DM	24	89	0.0293 ± 0.0029	194

Source: modified from Rosenqvist et al. (1976), p 583, table 2, with permission from The American Diabetes Association

space (Table 2-2). Giddings et al. (1977) reported glucose space calculated from volume in which glucose load would have been diluted to achieve the observed plasma glucose concentrations at 3 min from the start of continuous glucose infusion (0.167 mg/kg min). Although the actual volume was not described in their report, they found a decrease in the distribution volume of 1.24 l on the first operative day as compared with preoperative values in 18 elective abdominal surgical patients.

Our Early Studies

We had been studying insulin response and glucose clearance during various types of anesthesia in mongrel dogs (Ishihara et al. 1981). We also had been studying acute insulin response (AIR) during and immediately after general anesthesia and gynecological abdominal surgery in which 25 ml 20% glucose (5 g) was administered intravenously over 30 s and blood samples were obtained immediately before injection and at 3, 5, and 10 min postinjection by repeated arterial punctures (Ishihara et al. 1985). In this study, the effect of an infusion of the ganglion blocking agent trimetaphan (15 μg/kg min), which would modify AIR through suppression of norepinephrine release, was studied. AIR was evaluated by using the mean incremental plasma insulin concentration at 3 and 5 min postinjection above the preinjection value. AIR was decreased to 15.7% during surgery and further to 9.7% after surgery compared with preanesthetic values in the absence of a trimetaphan infusion, whereas it was decreased only to 43.9% during surgery and further to 23.9% after surgery in the presence of a trimetaphan infusion. There was a statistical difference with or without a trimetaphan infusion ($P < 0.01$, respectively) (Fig. 2-1).

Assuming that AIR plays a major role in determining incremental plasma glucose levels shortly after glucose challenge, the magnitude of incremental plasma glucose levels would consistently be increased when AIR is suppressed. In contrast, the magnitude would be associated less with a trimetaphan infusion compared with no trimetaphan infusion. However, these changes based on AIR response were not actually observed during and after surgery in our study. Although the magnitude of incremental plasma glucose concentrations at 3 min postinjection were obviously increased during surgery by an average of 16.3 mg/100 ml compared with that before induction of anesthesia, the postoperative magnitude returned to that before induction of anesthesia (Fig. 2-2).

A trimetaphan infusion failed to decrease the magnitude of incremental plasma glucose levels but conversely increased the magnitude of incremental plasma glucose levels despite augmented acute insulin response, suggesting that AIR has no significant impact on the magnitude of incremental plasma

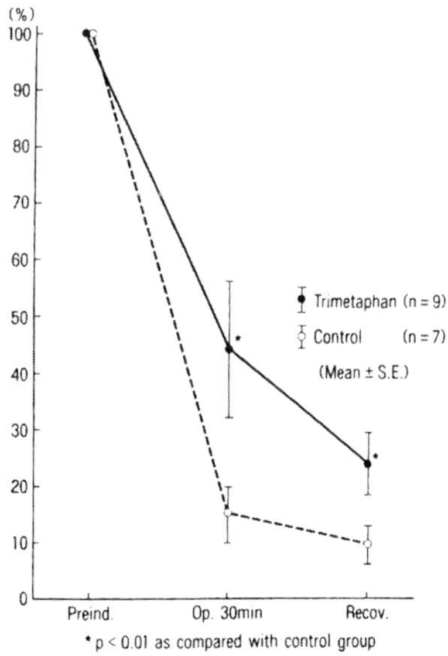

FIG. 2-1. Acute insulin response following surgery. *Preind.*, preinduction of anesthesia; *Op.*, during operation; *Recov.*, when patients had recovered adequately from anesthesia in the recovery room. *$P < 0.01$ as compared with control group. (From Ishihara et al. (1985), p 628, fig. 2, with permission from Kokuseidoh)

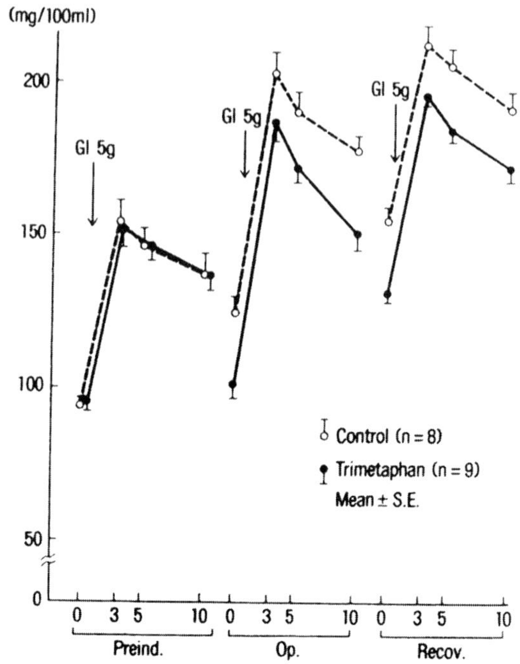

FIG. 2-2. Plasma glucose level following surgery. *Preind.*, preinduction of anesthesia; *Op.*, during operation; *Recov.*, when patients had recovered adequately from anesthesia in the recovery room. (From Ishihara et al. (1986b), p 1058, fig. 1, with permission from Kokuseidoh)

glucose levels early after glucose challenge, even though both intraoperative and postoperative actual plasma glucose levels before glucose challenge were significantly lower in trimetaphan-treated patients than those without it ($P < 0.01$). These results convincingly allowed us to explore the utility of glucose as an indicator for dilution volumetry other than the utility of glucose as a nutritional substance.

Glucose space in our early study was calculated using a one-compartment model from incremental plasma glucose levels using 3, 5, and 10 min postinfusion (Ishihara et al. 1986b). Preanesthetic glucose space was 7.0 ± 1.5 (SD) l (135 ± 21 ml/kg) in patients without a trimetaphan infusion and 8.1 ± 1.7 l (156 ± 53 ml/kg) in those with a trimetaphan infusion (Fig. 2-3). These values without a trimetaphan infusion were decreased to 77% of the preanesthetic value during surgery and returned to the preanesthetic value after surgery, whereas these values with a trimetaphan infusion were decreased to 56% and 77% of the preanesthetic value during and after surgery, respectively. Considering these findings, an infusion of trimetaphan yields a consistent decrease in glucose space. Redistribution of blood flow from the highly per-

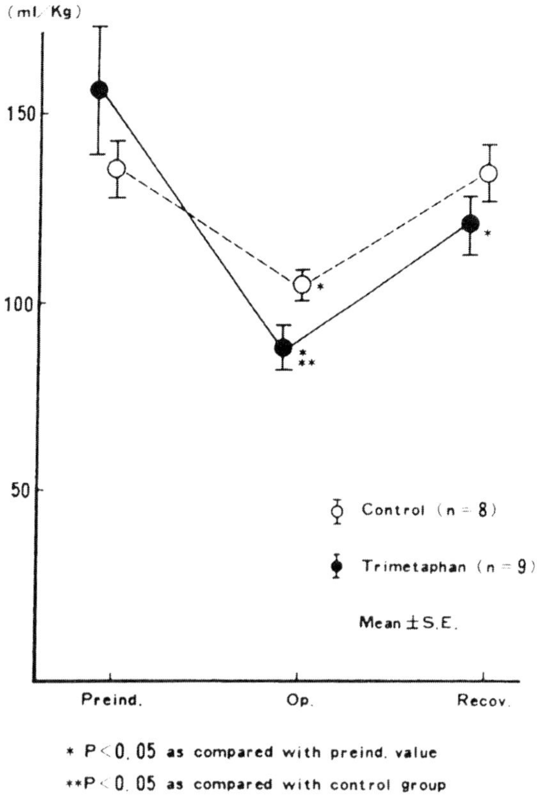

FIG. 2-3. Changes of glucose space following anesthesia and surgery. *Preind.*, preinduction of anesthesia; *Op.*, during operation; *Recov.*, when patients had recovered adequately from anesthesia in the recovery room. *$P < 0.05$ as compared with preind. value; **$P < 0.05$ as compared with control group. (From Ishihara et al. (1986b), p 1059, fig. 2, with permission from Kokuseidoh)

fused mesenteric vessels to the peripheral blood beds including skin and muscles (Wang et al. 1977) would be responsible for the decrease. Consequently, glucose space has potential of being an alternative measure of highly perfused fluid volume in the body without apparent modification by glucose metabolism, even though the sampling period and the procedure of our early study are not exactly same as those of currently performed measurements.

After our early study, we used insulinogenic index as a measure of insulin response to a glucose load in our early experimental studies (Shimodate et al. 1994, 1995) to evaluate the contribution of insulin on glucose metabolism. The index was calculated by dividing the area circumscribed by the plasma insulin–time curve (i.e., the incremental area above the level before a glucose administration) by the plasma glucose–time curve throughout the corresponding sampling period (Seltzer et al. 1967). No significant correlation was found between glucose space and the insulinogenic index before and after experimental hemorrhage, supporting the negligible effect of insulin response on glucose space. Furthermore, we did not take into account the urinary loss of glucose, because our previous report (Ishihara et al. 1981) demonstrated that urinary loss of glucose did not exceed 4.5% of the administered glucose during 60 min after glucose challenge, even when a relatively large glucose dose (0.5 g/kg) was administered.

Criticism of Our Experimental Study

Hahn (1996) commented on our glucose space study, which showed a decrease in glucose space following hemorrhagic shock (Shimodate et al. 1995). According to his comments, the hyperglycemic effect of hemorrhagic shock is likely to impose certain limitations on the usefulness of glucose space. Hemorrhage mobilizes glucose by means of gluconeogenesis, and the glucose level may double or, if glycogen stores are filled, even triple. In the cat and in the rat, this effect is fully developed within 1 h after a severe bleeding event. A progressive increase in endogenous blood glucose acts to decrease glucose space. Although we did not observe any extremely high plasma glucose level (>250 mg/100 ml) during hemorrhagic hypotension, augmented endogenous glucose output from the liver may have a significant impact on determination of glucose space.

Response to the Criticism

Assuming that the hyperglycemia that is present before a glucose challenge is a guide to endogenous glucose production, no correlation was found between glucose space and the preinjection plasma glucose concentration in our glucose space studies, including hemorrhagic shock (Shimodate et al. 1994; Koh et al. 1995). In addition, the rate of glucose disappearance from the plasma after glucose challenge (Ke-glucose) has been reported to slow in accordance with the magnitude of the hyperglycemia present before its injection (Wolfe et al. 1978), which may also be expected to modify the measurement of glucose space. However, no correlation was found between the preinjection plasma glucose concentration and Ke-glucose in our glucose space studies during hemorrhage and volume challenge (Koh et al. 1995; Miyahara et al. 1995). From these observations it would appear that hyperglycemic modification can be negligible during a short period after glucose challenge (Ishihara 1996c). Considering the amount of glucose load and sampling timing of our glucose studies, our glucose study stood in contrast to traditional glucose challenge studies previously described.

In 2005, Hahn again commented on our report regarding approximation of glucose space only using two blood samples: preinjection and 3 min postinjection (Ishihara et al. 2005a). His comment was that "Such simplification is justified because variations in glucose clearance and endogenous glucose production are of little importance near short time increments, at least when it is applied in a fairly coherent group of patients." Contribution of glucose metabolism on the distribution volume of glucose is discussed in more detail in the next chapter.

3. Models of Glucose Distribution and Utilization

Radioisotopic studies support the negligible effects of glucose metabolism during the early period after glucose administration, and glucose metabolism would have no obvious impact on initial distribution volume of glucose (IDVG) measurement.

Models Proposed by Cobelli's Group

Glucose intravenously administered equilibrates very rapidly with a volume greater than circulating blood volume. Although a one-compartment model was previously applied to calculate glucose space, it ignores the heterogenicity of glucose kinetics. Models for glucose distribution and utilization in man contain at least two glucose pools, one of which turns over slowly. The other, the fast pool, is divided into blood and the extravascular spaces, as described by Cobelli's group (Cobelli et al. 1990) (Fig. 3-1).

Cobelli's group has further proposed a three-compartment model. The fast pool consists of plasma and the extravascular space of highly perfused tissues (average rate of exchange with plasma, 1.09 ± 0.15/min). The slow pool consists of muscles and adipose tissues where exchanges are tenfold slower (average rate of exchange, 0.12 ± 0.01/min). The IDVG is identical to the plasma pool (40 ± 3 mg/kg, 46 ml/kg); the other fast and slow compartments have similar size (91 ± 12 mg/kg, 104 ml/kg and 96 ± 9 mg/kg, 110 ml/kg) (Fig. 3-2). Accordingly, the total distribution volume of glucose in the basal state is 260 ± 5 ml/kg.

Glucose Uptake

Administered glucose is rapidly taken up into cells of the cerebral, splanchnic, renal medulla, and erythrocytes by facilitated diffusion, but insulin is not. The cumulative glucose uptake in these tissues in the basal state can

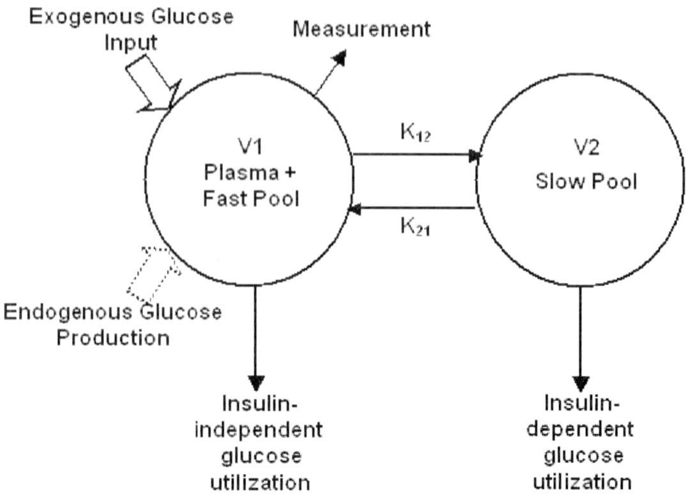

FIG. 3-1. The two-compartment model of whole-body glucose distribution and disposal. (Modified from Cobelli et al. Horm Metab Res 1990;24(suppl):1–10, p 4, fig. 6)

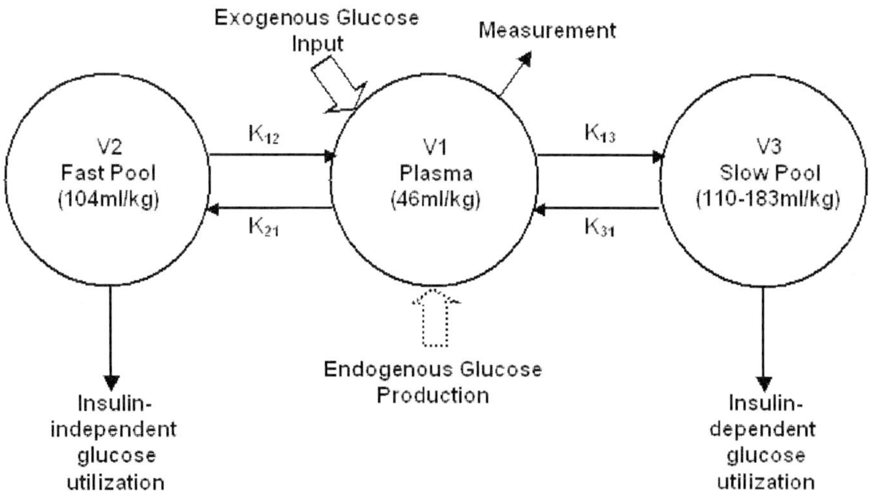

FIG. 3-2. The three-compartment model of whole-body glucose distribution and disposal based on the concept proposed by Cobelli's group (Ferrannini et al. J Clin Invest 1985;76:357–364; Cobelli et al. 1990;24(suppl):1–10; modified from p 2, fig. 3). Insulin administration yields a marked increase in the size of the slow pool

TABLE 3-1. Summary of blood flow and glucose uptake rates by intact organs of human in the basal postabsorptive state

	Blood flow (ml/kg min)	Blood flow (% of cardiac output)	Glucose uptake (mg/kg min)	Glucose uptake (% of total)
Brain	12	15	1.2	55
Splanchnic organs	21	26	0.5	23
Kidneys	16	20	<0.1	<1
Muscle	13	16	0.3	14
Heart	2	3	0.09	4
Erythrocytes	—	—	0.06	3
Other	16	20	<0.01	<1
Total	80	100	2.2	100

Source: modified from Ferrannini et al. (1985), p 361, table 2, with permission from J Clin Invest

be estimated as 1.5–1.7 mg/kg min or 75% of basal glucose uptake (Table 3-1) (Ferrannini et al. 1985). Consequently, the fast pool can be further identified as an insulin-independent pool. Neither the size nor the exchange rates of the plasma or the rapidly exchanging pool are appreciably changed, whereas glucose administered intravenously is slowly taken up into cells of muscle and adipose tissues by facilitated insulin (Ferrannini et al. 1985). Thus, the slow compartment can be identified as an insulin-dependent pool. Although interstitial glucose concentration in the adipose tissue increases only less than 50% of the maximal value during the first 7.5 min after intravenous bolus glucose injection, its maximum concentration occurs at 22 min after injection (Regittnig et al. 1999), suggesting that the extracellular mixing of intravenously injected glucose requires more than 22 min to be completed. Glucose uptake in the slow compartment reaches to 83% of total glucose uptake during insulin administration, and at the same time the size of the slow pool is markedly expanded (to 190 ± 30 mg/kg), and furthermore, total glucose uptake rises fourfold of basal values (to 7.96 mg/kg min). In contrast, Youn et al. (1995) reported that insulin does not affect extracellular glucose distribution kinetics in conscious rats. Steil et al. (1996) demonstrated that insulin does not increase transcapillary glucose diffusion to insulin-sensitive cells. These findings would at least allow speculation that insulin does not have a significant impact on the size of the fast pool.

As the results of radioisotopic studies did not support the appreciable contribution of glucose metabolism to its pharmacokinetic disposition for a short period after glucose challenge (Ferrannini et al. 1985), plasma glucose data during the first 8 min postinjection have not been used for evaluation of either glucose uptake or suppression of glucose production (Vicini et al. 1997).

Irreversible Loss of Administered Glucose

Irreversible loss of administered glucose into urine and the brain rather than insulin-dependent tissues can be assumed.

Urinary Loss of Glucose

Glycosuria will occur when plasma glucose concentration is greater than 256 mg/100 ml in humans, equivalent to an arterial whole blood glucose concentration of 2.2 mg/ml (Cunningham and Heath 1978). The mean glomerular filtration rate during urinary loss of glucose is equivalent to 2.1 ml blood (ml/kg min). Thus, renal glucose loss is as follows:

$$R = 2.1 \times (0.01 \times C - 2.2)$$

where R = renal glucose loss (mg/min/kg) and C = arterial whole blood glucose concentration (mg/100 ml).

Presumably, urinary loss of administered glucose would appear to be negligible in a short period after a small amount of glucose (5 g) injection, even if subsequent transient hyperglycemia (>220 mg/100 ml) is developed in normal kidney function. We found that urinary loss of glucose does not exceed 4.5% of the glucose load (0.5 g/kg) during 60 min postinjection in experimental canine study (Ishihara et al. 1981). Additionally, urine output remained less than 10 ml/kg during 60 min even after 30 ml/kg fluid volume challenge in an experimental canine study (Miyahara et al. 1995). Considering these findings, we did not take into account the urinary loss of glucose in our glucose space study.

Glucose Uptake in the Brain

Glucose uptake is thought to be 1.08 mg/kg min (Insel et al. 1975) and is substantially independent of blood glucose or insulin concentrations (Cunningham and Heath 1978). Presumably, glucose uptake remains unchanged during the sampling period of our glucose space study.

Hepatic Glucose Output and Uptake

Hepatic glucose output is reported to be maintained at a rate of 2 mg/kg min in man (Insel et al. 1975). In normal humans, glucose administration rapidly inhibits hepatic glucose output (Cunningham and Heath 1978). Complete inhibition will develop immediately after the start of injection. Furthermore, hepatic glucose uptake can occur during the subsequent sampling period, even though the magnitude of the uptake is less in intravenous glucose administration as compared with oral administration. In diabetic patients

TABLE 3-2. Effect of hepatic glucose output during intravenous glucose tolerance test on glucose space in diabetic patients

	Output (+)	Output (–)
Nonobese, mild diabetic	237 ml/kg	236 ml/kg
Obese, mild diabetic	221 ml/kg	218 ml/kg
Nonobese, moderate diabetes	254 ml/kg	253 ml/kg

(+), Glucose production was maintained throughout the test; (–), glucose production was suppressed completely throughout the test

Source: modified from Cunningham and Heath (1978), p 168, table 4, with permission from the Medical Research Socity and the Biochemical Society

and critically ill patients such as trauma, burn, or septic patients, suppression of hepatic glucose output is less pronounced or unchanged following glucose injection (Cunningham and Heath 1978). It is unclear that hepatic glucose output is suppressed or unchanged during the sampling period in each individual patient, which may affect the result of our glucose space. However, the cumulative glucose space remains unchanged whether or not hepatic glucose output is assumed during the procedure (Table 3-2).

4. Glucose Dilution in Practice

In the previous chapters, we used the term glucose space for the distribution volume of glucose. From this chapter on, we advocate initial distribution volume of glucose (IDVG) instead, because our glucose space does not cover the entire glucose distribution but rather its initial distribution phase only. Original measurement of our IDVG requires repeated blood sampling throughout 7 min postinjection and applying a one-compartment model to the incremental values above preinjection. In this chapter, the measurement procedure of original IDVG, its normal value, its repeatability, and its approximation are described.

Patient Selection

We have performed more than 4000 IDVG determinations, not only for research purposes but also as a routine clinical variable for point-of-care testing in most of our intensive care unit (ICU) patients. We did not experience any adverse sequelae from IDVG determinations. Exclusion criteria for IDVG determinations include the presence of excessive hyperglycemia and/or central nervous system ischemia. Although the result of IDVG determination is not appreciably modified by the magnitude of hyperglycemia present before glucose challenge (maximal limits, 300 mg/100 ml according to our experience), sustained hyperglycemia itself has been recognized to alter the outcome of critically ill patients. Thus, we should be concerned about normalization of basal blood glucose levels (less than 150 mg/100 ml is desirable). Additionally, changes in the infusion rate of a glucose-containing solution immediately before or during blood sampling should be avoided. We have performed IDVG determinations even during fluid resuscitation and hemodynamically unstable states, such as during fluid resuscitation for burned patients. According to our experience, IDVG determinations even in such critical conditions are still useful for therapeutic decision making for critically ill patients.

Determination of IDVG

In our early studies, an infusion of 25 ml glucose 20% (5 g) was given over 30 s through a central venous line. Currently, a bolus injection of 10 ml, 50% (5 g) is used instead. Serial blood samples were obtained through an indwelling artery catheter, immediately before and 3, 4, 5, and 7 min after glucose administration. Isotonic saline with small amounts of heparin was used to flush the lines after each sampling and glucose injection. A glucose-containing solution for routine fluid and nutritional management remains unchanged throughout the procedures.

Model Selection for IDVG Determination

We have been applying a one-compartment model to calculate IDVG, although this simplest model has been indicated as a possible source of error for describing complete pharmacokinetic disposition (Ferrannini et al. 1985; Regittnig et al. 1999). Furthermore, the normal value of our IDVG is greater than plasma volume, and closer to the combined plasma and rapidly exchanging pool volumes. Plasma concentration at 1 min postinjection would be apparently influenced even in a small variability of blood sampling time and the injection procedure because the magnitude of decay in the increased plasma glucose concentration around 1 min postinjection is apparently greater compared to 3 min postinjection or thereafter. Thus, we do not use values at 1 min postinjection but at 3 min postinjection to ensure complete mixing within the central compartment. As judged by the observed value at 3 min postinjection, intravenously administered glucose has been already distributed not only within plasma but also into the extravascular rapidly exchanging compartment. Consequently, our IDVG would not indicate the true initial distribution volume of glucose, namely plasma volume, proposed by Cobelli's group (Cobelli et al. 1990), but rather the fast pool volume as a whole, namely, total volumes of plasma and the extravascular rapid exchanging compartment. Considering that IDVG generally has more than twofold plasma volume and that circulating time of blood is not uniform among tissues (Hoeft et al. 1994), the size of the extravascular rapid exchanging compartment rather than the plasma volume has a major impact on IDVG.

As the glucose load in our study is smaller than that in the conventional intravenous glucose challenge test, some ICU patients failed to show a consistent decrease in plasma glucose concentrations for the first 30 min following 5 g intravenous glucose administration (Ishihara et al. 1998b). Additionally, more than 30 min is required to analyze the entire plasma decay curve, even using a two-compartment model (Cunningham and Heath 1978). Considering these observations, a one-compartment model was used for plasma glucose data up to 7 min postinfusion in the IDVG study, even though IDVG calculated using a one-compartment model overestimated that of a two-compartment model by an average of 0.57 ± 0.66 l in our clinical study (Ishihara et al. 1998b).

We have observed a decline of plasma glucose concentrations throughout 60 min postinjection, even though plasma glucose concentrations at 60 min postinjection remained elevated slightly compared with the preinjection value in hemodynamically stable patients (Rose et al. 2004). Although IDVG measurement would not induce a prolonged hyperglycemic state even in critically ill patients, and some evidence exists that transient hyperglycemia is not harmful, we should be concerned about normalization of basal plasma glucose concentration rather than a transient hyperglycemia in these patients. Diaz-Parejo et al. (2003) suggest that transient moderate hyperglycemia has no adverse effect on outcome in patients with severe traumatic brain lesions and stroke.

Evaluation of Glucose Decay Curve

IDVG is determined using a least squares regression technique to find the line of the best fit. A nonlinear multiple regression program (MULTI) is used (Yamaoka et al. 1981, 1985). Akaike's information criterion (AIC) (Akaike 1985) is examined to evaluate the exponential term of the pharmacokinetic model as follows:

$$\mathrm{AIC} = -N \times \ln(\mathrm{SSQ_w}) + 2\mathrm{P}$$

where N = the number of data points, $\mathrm{SSQ_w}$ = the residual sum of squares, and P = the number of parameters identified in the model. AIC is originally designed to evaluate the adequacy of the selected model. Because low AIC values indicate a superiority of fitness between the observed data points and the regression curve, we have been using AIC in our IDVG study to evaluate fitness of the IDVG curve, even though we only apply a one-compartment model for calculation of IDVG (Fig. 4-1).

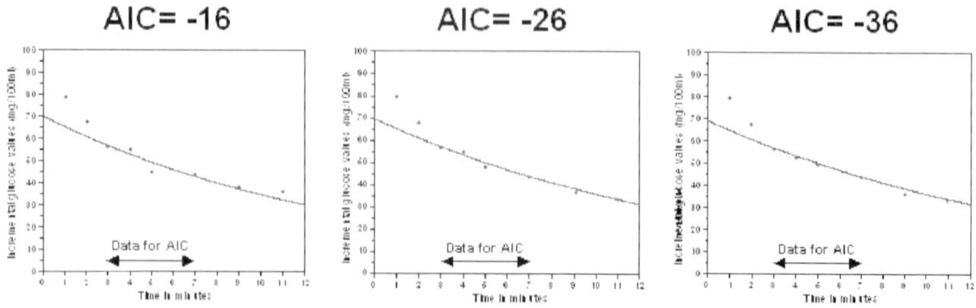

FIG. 4-1. Various Akaike's information criterion (AIC) values and the fitness between initial distribution volume of glucose (IDVG) curve and data points. Regression line and AIC are determined using four incremental postinjection values: 3, 4, 5, and 7 min postinjection

Normal IDVG Values

Normal IDVG values were determined in 16 healthy volunteers, mostly medical students, regardless of fasting state (Table 4-1). Normal IDVG values were also calculated as 105–142 ml/kg from the reported normal plasma volume derived by the ICG dilution method (PV-ICG) of 40–50 ml/kg in humans (Sekimoto et al. 1997) and the PV-ICG/IDVG ratio of 0.35–0.38 based on our study (Ishihara et al. 1999). Additionally, in our earlier experimental canine study, the normovolemic IDVG was 117–124 ml/kg (Iwakawa et al. 1998; Suzuki et al. 1999). Considering these findings, the normal IDVG range is approximately from 110 to 130 ml/kg.

IDVG in our 16 volunteers ranged from 97 to 130 ml/kg or 3.3 to 4.8 l/m^2 with or without overnight fasting (Table 4-1). The mean IDVG was 112 ± 12 ml/kg or 4.0 ± 0.5 l/m^2. The value is relatively smaller compared with IDVG reported in our first glucose study in 16 gynecological surgical patients immediately before induction of anesthesia of 135–156 ml/kg (Ishihara et al. 1986b). The latter patients had no arterial line to draw blood samples; each arterial blood sample was obtained using repeated arterial punctures instead. Additionally, the sampling timing was extended to 10 min postinjection in the latter instead of 7 min postinjection in the former. Thus, glucose metabolism may play a role at least partly in determining plasma glucose concentration at 10 min postinjection. Furthermore, the arterial puncture method would be less accurate to obtain punctual sample timing. Presumably, these different sampling procedures might affect the result of IDVG in our early IDVG study.

IDVG in Critically Ill Patients

Although normal IDVG values are presented in this chapter, optimal fluid volume status may vary with each individual patient as well as with the underlying pathology. According to our experience with more than 4000

TABLE 4-1. Initial distribution volume of glucose in 16 volunteers

No.	Sex	Age (years)	Height (cm)	BW (kg)	BSA (/m²)	Hct (%)	TP (g/100 ml)	pre-inj (mg/100 ml)	3 min (mg/100 ml)	4 min (mg/100 ml)	5 min (mg/100 ml)	7 min (mg/100 ml)	AIC	Ke-gl (/min)	IDVG (l)	IDVG[a] (ml/kg)	IDVG[b] (l/m²)
1	M	55	167	60	1.67	38.3	6.8	89	52	47	46	38	−21.8	0.0755	7.69	128	4.60
2	M	28	170	65	1.75	38.5	6.8	99	48	43	40	35	−24.8	0.076	8.42	130	4.81
3	M	24	180	74	1.93	50.9	8.0	94	42	38	36	31	−27.5	0.0738	9.64	130	4.99
4	M	29	164	52	1.55	47.3	6.5	94	74	64	60	40	−22.3	0.094	5.21	100	3.36
5	M	22	171	67.5	1.79	45.1	7.6	85	55	52	45	38	−22.5	0.0959	6.75	100	3.77
6	F	25	151	44	1.36	40	6.8	92	73	67	62	54	−31.7	0.074	5.51	125	4.05
7	M	22	168	68	1.77	41.9	6.5	92	62	55	52	48	−19.8	0.060	6.96	102	3.93
8	M	23	171	62	1.73	42	6.8	87	64	57	52	44	−26.9	0.092	6.00	97	3.47
9	M	25	180	68	1.86	44	6.8	99	54	47	43	34	−27.1	0.1135	6.65	98	3.57
10	F	22	168	53	1.59	33.4	6.2	88	72	67	61	55	−25.2	0.067	5.71	108	3.59
11[c]	M	25	183	72	1.93	41.4	7.0	116	54	53	47	45	−19.5	0.049	7.98	111	4.14
12[c]	M	24	184	67	1.88	46.3	6.2	124	49	44	40	34	−28.0	0.0905	7.85	117	4.18
13[c]	F	23	164.7	51.5	1.55	38.6	6.4	102	81	71	68	60	−20.8	0.0705	5.14	100	3.32
14[c]	M	25	179	69	1.87	35.6	6.8	132	48	42	39	34	−21.5	0.0829	8.34	121	4.46
15[c]	M	25	177	72	1.89	42.7	6.6	99	52	46	43	39	−20.4	0.0686	8.07	112	4.27
16[c]	M	24	168	63	1.72	40.1	6.3	184	58	53	49	45	−22.6	0.0623	7.29	116	4.24
Mean		26	172	63	2	41.6	6.8	105	59	53	49	42	−23.9	0.078	7.08	112	4.05
SD		8	9	9	0	4.5	0.5	25	11	10	9	9	3.5	0.016	1.31	12	0.51

For plasma glucose levels and IDVG in each individual volunteer, the plasma glucose levels present before glucose challenge ranged from 88 to 184 mg/100 ml; AIC for glucose decay curve ranged from −19.4 to −31.7, indicating each glucose decay curve is adequately fitted as shown in Fig. 4-1

BW, body weight; BSA, body surface area; Hct, hematocrit; TP, total plasma protein; preinj., plasma glucose before injection; AIC, Akaike's information criterion; Ke-gl, disappearance rate of increased plasma glucose concentrations; IDVG, initial distribution volume of glucose

[a]Based on body weight

[b]Based on body surface area

[c]After food intake

TABLE 4-2. Pharmacokinetic variables in the 30- and 60-min groups

	30-min group		60-min group	
	0 min	30 min	0 min	60 min
GL (mmol/l)	7.9 (2.1; 2.7–11.2)	9.2 (2.3; 3.0–13.1)	7.7 (2.1; 5.3–12.3)	9.0** (3.0; 6.4–17.3)
AIC	–23.84 (3.58; –18.61) to –31.46)	–23.58 (4.83; –12.46 to –34.75)	–24.46 (4.15; –17.16 to –33.27)	–23.57 (7.04; –14.69 to –41.39
IDVG (l)	6.69 (0.96; 5.43–9.07)	6.77 (1.03; 5.28–8.56)	7.17 (2.05; 5. 23–11.30)	6.98 (1.97; 5.15–10.43)
Ke-gl (/min)	0.071 (0.012; 0.052–0.096)	0.081* (0.015; 0.055–0.102)	0.069 (0.013; 0.050–0.096)	0.084 (0.026; 0.044–0.123)

Values are presented as mean (SD; range)
GL, plasma glucose level before injection; AIC, Akaike's information criterion (6); IDVG, initial distribution volume of glucose; Ke-gl, glucose disappearence rate from plasma
*$P < 0.001$; **$P = 0.011$
Source: from Rose et al. (2004), p 320, table 3, with permission from Blackwell

IDVG measurements in the ICU, some patient groups require a greater fluid volume to stabilize their hemodynamic state. Patients with chronic renal failure or hepatic failure had a larger IDVG than normal. In contrast, obese patients had a relatively smaller IDVG than nonobese patients based on their total body weight. Presumably, lean body mass would be preferable as the basal body weight for evaluation of IDVG in obese patients. Thus, optimal fluid volume status for each underlying pathology is a subject that needs future investigation.

Repeatability of IDVG Determination

To assess the repeatability of IDVG determination, 29 ICU patients were studied. After achieving a hemodynamically stable state in each patient regardless of an infusion of vasoactive drugs, two glucose challenges at an interval of either 30 or 60 min were carried out to calculate IDVG (Rose et al. 2004). Although plasma glucose concentrations immediately before the second glucose challenge in either group were higher than those immediately before the first challenge ($P < 0.001$, respectively), the bias of IDVG measurements was 0.08 ± 0.321 (1.2% ± 3.9%) for the 30-min group and –0.19 ± 0.281 (–2.6% ± 7.8%) for the 60-min group (Figs. 4-2, 4-3; see Table 4-2). An increase in the basal plasma glucose level present before the second glucose challenge did not alter IDVG in our patients in either group. Results indicate that IDVG determinations can be reliably repeated within a minimum interval of 30 min.

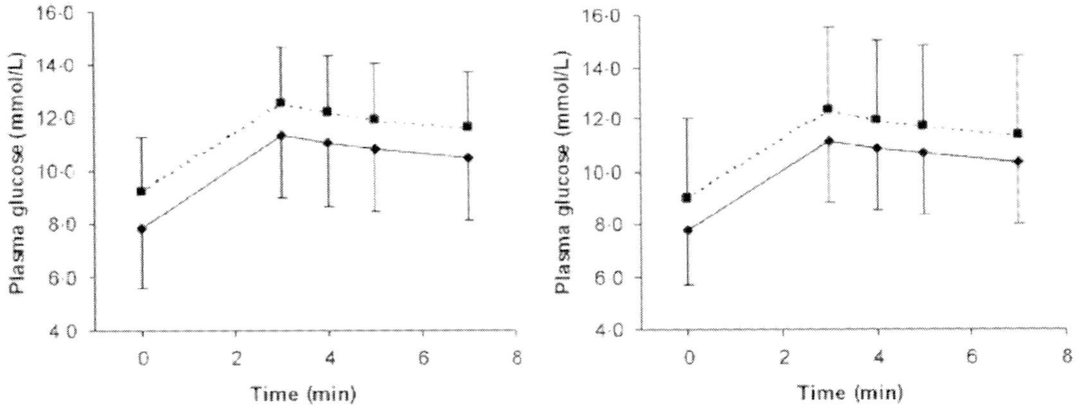

FIG. 4-2. Course of plasma glucose concentration after the first (*solid line*) and second (*dashed line*) glucose injection presented as mean and SD. *Left*, 30-min group; *right*, 60-min group. (From Rose et al. (2004), p 320, fig. 1, with permission from Blackwell)

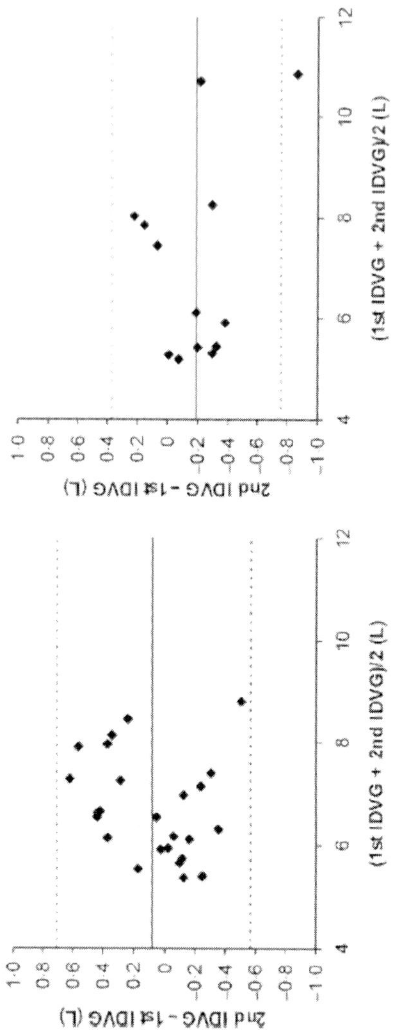

Fig. 4-3. Agreement between first and second IDVG measurement shown by Bland and Altman plots (*solid line*, mean difference; *dashed lines*, ±2 SD). *Left*, 30-min group; right, 60-min group, −0.19 ± 0.561 (−2.6% ± 7.8%). (From Rose et al. (2004), p 320, fig. 2, with permission from Blackwell)

van Tulder et al. (2005) reported weak reproducibility of IDVG determination soon after cardiac surgery. According to their report, however, their patients might have internal bleeding, temperature change, alterations in vasomotor tone, or fluid shifts between compartments during the repeated measurements of IDVG, even though routine clinical monitoring supported stable hemodynamic states. Junghans et al. (2002) demonstrated that clinical judgments about the patient's intravascular volume based on conventional monitoring even by experienced physicians are absolutely contrary to those based on measurement of intrathoracic blood volume (ITBV) after upper gastrointestinal tract surgery. Thus, patients early after cardiac surgery would not be good candidates for evaluation of the repeatability of IDVG determination (Ishihara 2006). Considering their unstable hemodynamic state, cardiac surgical patients whose postoperative admittance to the ICU was less than 12h before glucose challenge were excluded from our repeatability study (Rose et al. 2004).

Approximation of IDVG

Measurement of IDVG originally required repeated arterial blood sampling throughout 7min after glucose injection. To reduce both turnaround time and the amount of blood samples, we proposed a simplified formula using only two blood samples: immediately before glucose injection and at 3min after injection. In the early IDVG studies we found a linear correlation between incremental plasma glucose concentration at 3min postinjection and IDVG (Ishihara et al. 1986a, 1993, 1998b):

$$\text{Approximated IDVG (l)} = -0.1 \times \Delta\text{Gl-3min (mg/100 ml)} + 13$$

where ΔGl-3min = incremental plasma glucose concentration at 3 min postinjection. IDVG can be approximated from one-point incremental plasma glucose concentration because the disappearance rate of glucose from plasma has a relatively small variability and remains relatively low, mostly ranging from 0.05/min to 0.10/min (average, 0.07/min). In contrast, the disappearance rate of indocyanine green (ICG) from plasma apparently varies among critically ill patients, ranging from 0.01/min to 0.35/min, resulting in failure of approximation of its distribution volume, namely, plasma volume, from the one-point plasma ICG concentration after injection.

The formula described above is very simple and clinically useful. As judged by plots of ΔGl-3 min and IDVG (Fig. 4-4), however, a good fit between approximated and original IDVGs seems unlikely when the incremental plasma glucose levels are either extremely high or low. Thus, we proposed

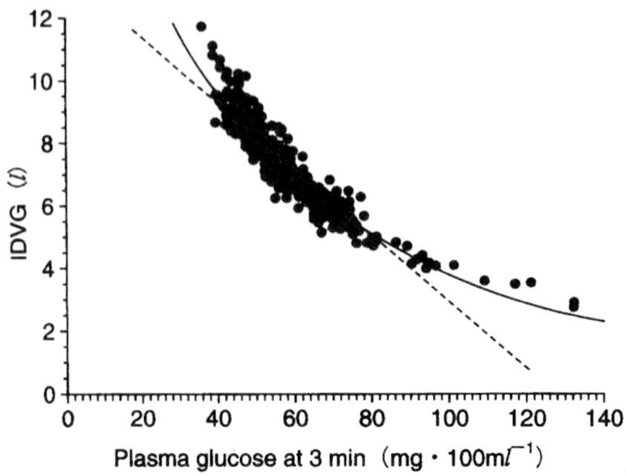

FIG. 4-4. Relationship between IDVG and incremental plasma glucose level at 3 min postinjection. *Solid regression curve* ($Y = 24.4\ e^{-0.03X} + 2.7$) (Hirota et al. 1999); *dashed regression line* ($Y = -0.1\ X + 13$) (Ishihara et al. 1998b). (From Ishihara (2000b), p 279, fig. 2-4, with permission from Kokuseidoh)

another formula using a one-phase exponential decay as follows (Hirota et al. 1999) (Table 4-3):

$$\text{Approximated IDVG(L)} = 24.4 \times e^{-0.03 \times \Delta \text{Gl-3min}} + 2.7$$

where ΔGl-3 min (mg/100 ml) = incremental plasma glucose concentration at 3 min postinjection. The agreement between approximated and measured IDVGs was assessed by Bland and Altman plots. The mean difference between the two volumes was −0.30 ± 0.43 l. Therefore, 95% confidence limits for agreement between the two volumes were from −0.88 l to 0.82 l (Fig. 4-5).

Approximation of IDVG Using a Conventional Glucose Analyzer

Although bedside reflectance glucometers rarely overestimate or underestimate the "true" glucose concentration by more than 40 mg/100 ml (2.2 mmol/l) (Ray et al. 2001), this margin of error is too great for measurement of IDVG. In addition, plasma protein concentrations, hematocrit, and body temperature, as well as blood oxygen tension, may influence measurements from such devices significantly (Maser et al. 1994; Karcher et al. 1993; Kurahashi et al. 1997). Accordingly, bedside glucometers were not used in our measurement of IDVG. Instead, we tested a conventional but more-accurate glucose analyzer (Ishihara et al. 2005a), specifically a combined blood gas and glucose analyzer, because many ICUs have this type of glucose analyzer, which would

TABLE 4-3. Approximated IDVG using incremental glucose level at 3 min postinjection

Δgl 3 min (mg/100 ml)	IDVG (l)	Δgl 3 min (mg/100 ml)	IDVG (l)	Δgl 3 min (mg/100 ml)	IDVG (l)
31	12.3	61	6.6	91	4.3
32	12.0	62	6.5	92	4.2
33	11.8	63	6.4	93	4.2
34	11.5	64	6.3	94	4.2
35	11.2	65	6.2	95	4.1
36	11.0	66	6.1	96	4.1
37	10.7	67	6.0	97	4.0
38	10.5	68	5.9	98	4.0
39	10.3	69	5.8	99	4.0
40	10.0	70	5.7	100	3.9
41	9.8	71	5.6	101	3.9
42	9.6	72	5.5	102	3.8
43	9.4	73	5.4	103	3.8
44	9.2	74	5.4	104	3.8
45	9.0	75	5.3	105	3.7
46	8.8	76	5.2	106	3.7
47	8.7	77	5.1	107	3.7
48	8.5	78	5.1	108	3.7
49	8.3	79	5.0	109	3.6
50	8.1	80	4.9	110	3.6
51	8.0	81	4.8	111	3.6
52	7.8	82	4.8	112	3.5
53	7.7	83	4.7	113	3.5
54	7.5	84	4.7	114	3.5
55	7.4	85	4.6	115	3.5
56	7.2	86	4.5	116	3.5
57	7.1	87	4.5	117	3.4
58	7.0	88	4.4	118	3.4
59	6.9	89	4.4	119	3.4
60	6.7	90	4.3	120	3.4

Each initial distribution volume of glucose (IDVG) was calculated using a formula we previously proposed (Hirota et al. 1999)

Δgl 3 min, increase in glucose concentration above the preinjection level at 3 min after injection

Source: from Ishihara et al. (2005a), p R146, table 2, with permission from Biomed Central

permit routine use of approximated IDVG as a measure of extracellular fluid volume in those units, provided that plasma or whole blood glucose concentrations measured using these devices are suitable for IDVG determination. A total of 50 patients admitted to the general ICU were included in this prospective study. Although patients may undergo several fluid volume determinations during their stay in the ICU, this study considered only the first

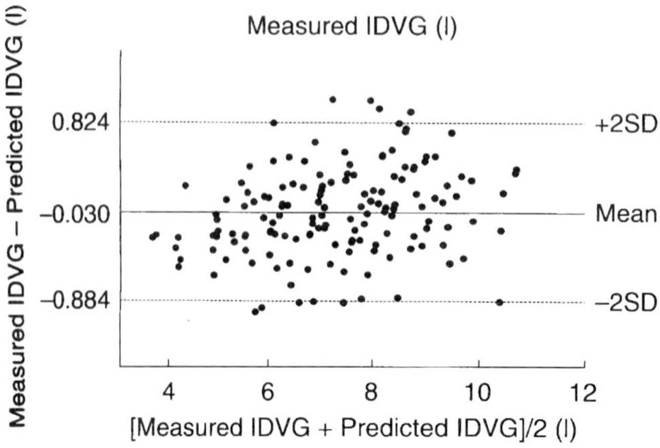

FIG. 4-5. Agreement between approximated and original IDVGs using Bland and Altman plots. (From Hirota et al. (1999), p 363, fig. 2 (lower part), with permission from Blackwell)

IDVG measurement in each patient during their stay in the ICU. Blood rather than plasma glucose measurement is clinically relevant in terms of time savings for measurement as well as a simple measurement procedure that does not require a centrifuge.

Both plasma and whole blood glucose concentrations were measured using a combined blood gas and glucose analyzer (EML100 radiometer; Electrolyte Metabolite Laboratory, Copenhagen, Denmark) from two blood samples: one drawn immediately before glucose injection and one at 3 min after injection. Other than automatic regular calibration, the analyzer was not calibrated. Plasma glucose concentrations in all blood samples were measured using amperometry by a glucose oxidase immobilized membrane-H_2O_2 electrode (glucose analyzer GA-1150; Arkray, Kyoto, Japan) as the reference. The interassay coefficients of variation were 2.6% for the former and 0.3% for the latter at a glucose concentration of 150 mg/100 ml ($n = 6$). Original IDVG (the reference) was calculated from the plasma decay curve with a one-compartment model from the increase above preinjection levels between 3 and 7 min postinjection, as described previously. Each approximated IDVG was calculated according to Table 4-3. Glucose concentrations and other variables for approximated IDVGs are shown in Table 4-4. Glucose concentrations in plasma were higher than in whole blood by an average of 2 ± 3 mg/100 ml ($P < 0.001$, $n = 100$). The mean hematocrit was 30.3% ± 5.5%, and total plasma protein concentration was 5.1 ± 0.7 g/100 ml. Neither hematocrit nor total plasma protein concentration had a correlation with differences of glucose values between plasma and whole blood samples.

TABLE 4-4. Glucose values and approximated IDVG

Variable	Reference[a]	Plasma[b]	Whole blood[b]
Preinjection glucose (mg/100 ml)	158 ± 42	155 ± 41	153 ± 40
Incremental glucose (mg/100 ml)[c]	58 ± 11	57 ± 12	57 ± 11
Difference in glucose (mg/100 ml)[d]	—	−2 ± 3	−3 ± 4
Approximated IDVG (l)	7.26 ± 1.73	7.38 ± 1.8	7.40 ± 1.65
Difference from original IDVG (ll)	−0.17 ± 0.47	−0.05 ± 0.54	−0.04 ± 0.62

Values are promoted as mean ± standard deviation
[a]From plasma glucose values using the same glucose analyzer for original IDVG
[b]Using a conventional glucose analyzer (combined blood gas and glucose analyzer) for approximated IDVG
[c]The incremental glucose value at 3 min after glucose injection
[d]Difference in glucose values in another plasma or whole blood from the reference plasma value
Source: from Ishihara et al. (2005a), p R147, table 3, with permission from Biomed Central

Bland and Altman plots of the differences between each approximated IDVG and original IDVG are shown in Fig. 4-6. There was a close correlation between each approximated IDVG and original IDVG ($r^2 = 0.94$, $P < 0.001$, $n = 50$ for the reference plasma values; $r^2 = 0.92$, $P < 0.001$, $n = 50$ for the plasma values from the conventional analyzer; and $r^2 = 0.89$, $n = 50$, $P < 0.001$ for whole blood from the conventional analyzer, respectively).

We reported that repeated IDVG measurements, done at an interval of 30 min, differ by 0.08 ± 0.32 l in hemodynamically stable patients (Rose et al. 2004). Based on this finding, the limits of clinical agreement for IDVG measurement can be set at ±0.4 l, although the limits within which the two methods were considered to be interchangeable were set at ±0.5 l/min for measurement of cardiac output (Zöllner et al. 2001). Although the difference between approximated and original IDVG in our study was not particularly great, it extended beyond the limits of agreement. Our previous study also showed that the difference between approximated and original IDVG was 0.03 ± 0.43 l in 150 paired data using the same reference plasma glucose measurement system (Hirota et al. 1999), again indicating that the methods are not interchangeable. However, bearing in mind the close correlation between the two measures and the clinically applicable measurement procedure for approximated IDVG, the latter is useful in the ICU.

Glucose rapidly traverses the red cell membrane by facilitated diffusion without requiring energy or insulin (Fogh-Andersen et al. 1990). Because the mass concentration of water in plasma is 0.93 kg H_2O/l and that in red cells is 0.71 kg H_2O/l, whole blood has a mass concentration of water

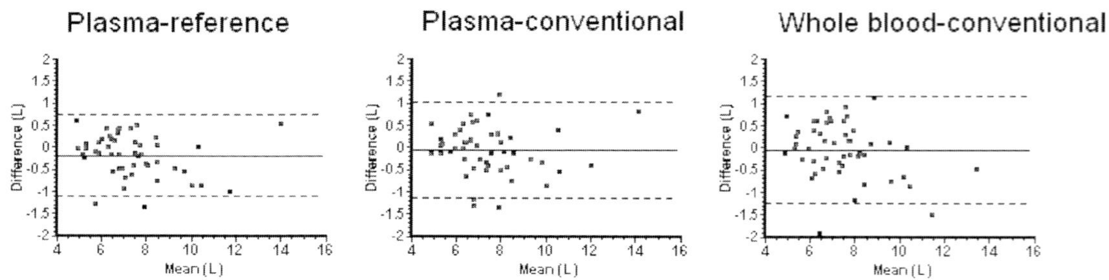

Fig. 4-6. Bland and Altman plots of the differences between each approximated IDVG and original IDVG. Approximated IDVG was calculated from a formula using the incremental glucose concentration (3) with the reference plasma glucose measurement (*left*), a conventional plasma glucose measurement (*middle*), and a conventional whole blood measurement (*right*). *Solid lines* represent the mean difference; *dashed lines* represent 95% confidence limits. (From Ishihara et al. (2005a), p R148, fig. 1, with permission from Biomed Central)

approximately 0.84 kg H_2O/l. Although the molality of glucose in plasma (mmol/kg H_2O) is equal in red cells, the glucose concentration in plasma (mmol/l) is higher than in either red cells or whole blood, depending on hematocrit of the blood sample (Fogh-Andersen et al. 1990). No significant correlation existed between hematocrit and the difference between paired plasma and whole blood glucose data in our study ($r^2 = 0.004$), but the plasma glucose value was significantly greater than that in whole blood. However, the impact of this difference on incremental value would be less significant than that on absolute values. Thus, we may approximate IDVG from two whole blood glucose measurements, even measurements determined using a conventional glucose analyzer (but not a bedside reflectance glucometer).

However, we believe that plasma glucose measurement is superior to whole blood glucose measurement, based on the bias and precision of our data as well as by the recommendation of plasma glucose rather than whole blood measurement (Kuwa et al. 2001). Furthermore, a 5%–10% decrease in whole blood glucose concentrations was observed during the first hour after sampling in routine condition (Savolainen et al. 1990). Whatever the calculation, it is important that all procedures must be performed using proper technique and accurate sampling time.

The turnaround time for approximated IDVG measurement from the first blood sample to completion of the calculation is about 5 min in our ICU. In our experience, gained by more than 4000 determinations of original IDVG, it can be measured during routine fluid management, and it is not necessary to stabilize plasma glucose concentrations, provided that the infusion rate of glucose for routine fluid management remains unchanged before and during the measurement procedure.

5. IDVG and Extracellular Fluid Volume

Although studies of glucose metabolism did not support the apparent modification of calculated results of initial distribution volume of glucose (IDVG) as described in the previous chapters, it remains unclear whether IDVG can mirror the central extracellular fluid (ECF) volume. We compared IDVG with the central ECF volume derived from sucrose dilution method in various volume states (Shimodate et al. 1995; Takamura et al. 1997; Iwakawa et al. 1998).

Sucrose as an Indicator of the ECF Volume

Since the 1930s, sucrose has been used in humans (Keith and Power 1937; Bauer et al. 1990) and animals (Raisz et al. 1953; Mulrow et al. 1956; White and Rolf 1958; Levin et al. 1970) for measuring ECF volume. Sucrose is better than inulin and sodium bromide because its low molecular weight (342) enables more even and rapid diffusion. In contrast to glucose, sucrose is little metabolized (Bauer et al. 1990). Less than 0.2% per minute of administered sucrose has been reported to be degraded in dogs (White and Rolf 1958).

Hemorrhagic Study

Eleven mongrel dogs weighing 7–9 kg were used for the study (Shimodate et al. 1995). Under pentobarbital anesthesia, mechanical ventilation with room air was continued throughout the experimental procedure. Glucose (100 mg/kg) and sucrose (400 mg/kg) were injected simultaneously over 30 s through the proximal port of the pulmonary artery catheter. Blood samples were drawn immediately before injection and during 120 min postinjection. Two hours later, blood was withdrawn at 1 ml/kg min for 30 min. At 30 min after completion of experimental hemorrhage, injection and blood sampling were repeated as previously. Plasma glucose concentrations were measured according to the glucose oxidase method (Gluco-20 glucose analyzer; Fuji, Tokyo, Japan), and plasma sucrose concentrations were determined using a spectrophotometric technique (U3200 spectrophotometer; Hitachi, Tokyo, Japan) by the method of Zweens and Frankena (1980). Plasma insulin concentrations were determined by radioimmunoassay (ARC-300, Aloka, Tokyo, Japan). The coefficient of variation of the measurement was less than 1% for glucose and 5% for sucrose.

To calculate the initial distribution volume of both glucose and sucrose (V_{dgluc} and V_{dsucr}, respectively), a one-compartment model was applied to excess or incremental plasma concentrations above basal values at 3–7 min after injection. The insulinogenic index, as described by Seltzer et al. (1967) was calculated by dividing the area enclosed by the plasma insulin–time curve (i.e., the incremental area above the level before injection) by the corresponding area enclosed by the plasma glucose–time curve throughout the 9-min sampling period.

The mean V_{dgluc} was 1.021 before hemorrhage and 0.761 after hemorrhage. The mean V_{dsucr} decreased from 0.911 to 0.631 and the mean insulinogenic index from 0.74 to 0.41 (Table 5-1). V_{dgluc} and V_{dsucr} were correlated ($r = 0.84$, $n = 22$, $P < 0.001$) (Fig. 5-1). However, there was no correlation between V_{dgluc} and the insulinogenic index ($r = 0.13$). V_{dgluc} overestimated V_{dsucr} by an average

TABLE 5-1. Distribution volumes and insulinogenic index before and after hemorrhage in mongrel dogs

No.	V_{dgluc}		V_{dsucr}		Insulinogenic index	
	Before	After	Before	After	Before	After
1	0.81	0.68	0.73	0.57	1.46	0.61
2	1.18	0.92	0.86	0.55	0.04	0.04
3	1.11	0.75	1.06	0.69	1.20	1.50
4	1.04	0.77	0.83	0.62	0.36	0.06
5	0.87	0.61	0.79	0.41	0.39	0.11
6	1.09	0.88	1.17	0.85	1.09	0.77
7	1.12	0.77	1.00	0.68	0.53	0.71
8	0.99	0.84	0.88	0.66	0.63	0.29
9	0.89	0.59	0.85	0.56	0.66	0.04
10	1.16	0.80	0.96	0.67	0.27	0.18
11	0.95	0.72	0.84	0.71	1.49	0.24
Mean	1.02	0.76	0.91	0.63	0.74	0.41
(SD)	(0.13)	(0.10)**	(0.13)	(0.11)**	(0.50)	(0.45)*

V_{dgluc}, initial distribution volume of glucose; V_{dsucr}, initial distribution volume of sucrose

* $P < 0.05$ vs. before; ** $P < 0.001$ vs. before

Source: from Shimodate et al. (1995), p 399, table 1, with permission from Cambridge University Press

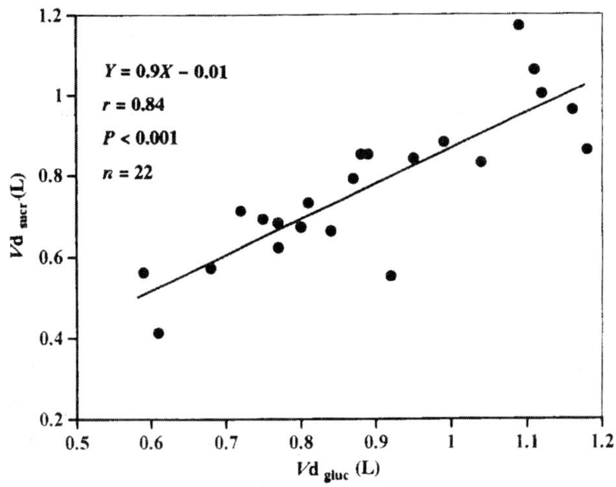

FIG. 5-1. Relationship between initial distribution volume of glucose (V_{dgluc}) and initial distribution volume of sucrose(V_{dsucr}). (From Shimodate et al. (1995), p 399, fig. 1, with permission from Cambridge University Press)

of 0.12 ± 0.10 l. Thus, the limits of agreement between the two methods were 0.32 l to −0.08 l. Thus, we conclude that glucose is equally effective as sucrose as a marker to measure ECF volume following hemorrhage.

Fluid Volume Loading Study

Ten mongrel dogs of either sex weighing 8.5–14.0 kg were used for this study (Takamura et al. 1997). Experimental preparation was essentially same as described in the hemorrhagic study. Glucose 100 mg/kg and sucrose 100 mg/kg were infused simultaneously through the proximal port of the pulmonary artery catheter over 30 s. Arterial samples were drawn immediately before and periodically during 30 min after the completion of infusion of the two indicators. Two hours later, the first fluid challenge was conducted with 3% low molecular weight dextran in lactated Ringer's solution, totaling 30 ml/kg over 30 min. Thirty minutes after the end of the fluid challenge, the second fluid challenge with the same amount of the dextran solution and the measurements and blood samplings were repeated as previously.

Low molecular weight dextran was administered for the fluid challenges in this study. However, sucrose cannot be distinguished from dextran in plasma by a spectrophotometric method. In a preliminary study, we administered 3% low molecular weight dextran in lactated Ringer's solution (30 ml/kg) over 30 min in three dogs to evaluate the effect of dextran on plasma sucrose concentration. The plasma sucrose concentration was 2.57 ± 0.42 mmol/l at 30 min after the end of the dextran infusion, when sucrose measurements were planned to start after each fluid challenge. The value remained unchanged during a short period thereafter: 2.67 ± 0.46 mmol/l at 3 min and 2.54 ± 0.54 mmol/l at 7 min thereafter. Presumably, the effect of dextran on sucrose measurements would have no apparent impact on the initial distribution volume of sucrose (IDVS) determination in this study, even though dextran in plasma can modify plasma sucrose concentration.

The mean prechallenge IDVG was 119.8 ± 12.1 ml/kg, which increased after the fluid challenge to 132.2 ± 6.7 ml/kg. The IDVG after the second challenge was 137.6 ± 22.1 ml/kg, even though a statistically significant difference was not obtained compared with the prechallenge value. The mean plasma sucrose concentration immediately before the second and the third infusions of sucrose was 2.51 ± 0.76 mmol/l and 3.44 ± 0.87 mmol/l, respectively. The mean Akaike's information criterion (AIC) was −18.6 ± 5.7 for IDVS determination. The mean prechallenge IDVS was 115.0 ± 13.8 ml/kg, which increased to 129.0 ± 11.9 ml/kg after the first challenge ($P < 0.02$). IDVS after the second fluid challenge was 137.4 ± 34.9 ml/kg, even though a statistically significant difference was not obtained compared with the prechallenge value (Table 5-2). Linear correlations were found between IDVG and IDVS ($r = 0.89$, $n = 28$, $P < 0.0001$) (Fig. 5-2) and between IDVG and cardiac output ($r = 0.48$, $n = 28$, $P < 0.02$). All dogs consistently showed that IDVG individually followed IDVS during changes in the latter. However, fluid challenges failed to consistently produce hypervolemia compared with prechallenge values. When examining whether there was an agreement between IDVG and IDVS, IDVG was found to exceed IDVS by an average of 2.9 ± 11.3 ml/kg. Therefore, the limits of agreement between the two volumes were −19.7 to +25.5 ml/kg. The urine output of nine of ten dogs was 13.0 ± 8.3 ml/kg between the first and the second infusions of the two indicators and 34.1 ± 12.8 ml/kg between the second and the third infusions. We conclude that glucose and sucrose were equally effective, and glucose was easier to measure because dextran interfered with sucrose determination.

Hemorrhagic and Subsequent Fluid Volume Loading Study

Twelve mongrel dogs of either sex weighing 8.0–12.0 kg were used (Iwakawa et al. 1998). Experimental preparation was same as performed in the previous study. In this study, we measured extravascular lung water (EVLW) as an indicator of extravascular fluid volume status in addition to the two fluid volumes. A lung water catheter (model HE-2900; Nihon Kohden, Tokyo,

Table 5-2. Distribution volumes and cardiac output in mongrel dogs

No.	Body weight (kg)	Initial distribution volume of glucose (ml/kg)			Initial distribution volume of sucrose (ml/kg)			Cardiac output (ml/kg min)		
		Prechallenge ($n = 10$)	First challenge ($n = 10$)	Second challenge ($n = 8$)	Prechallenge ($n = 10$)	First challenge ($n = 10$)	Second challenge ($n = 8$)	Prechallenge ($n = 10$)	First challenge ($n = 10$)	Second challenge ($n = 8$)
1	8.5	106.3	124.7	115.4	89.3	105.3	98.7	108.2	109.4	117.7
2	10.0	135.3	134.1	158.8	129.8	133.1	140.1	238.0	228.0	220.0
3	14.0	124.9	127.1	151.7	132.6	134.9	158.2	204.3	172.9	212.9
4	9.0	104.3	139.8	169.4	100.8	138.0	195.8	202.2	222.2	238.9
5	11.0	117.5	137.2	145.1	116.5	129.4	166.4	161.8	160.0	90.9
6	10.0	129.7	127.0	124.5	130.3	120.1	126.8	236.0	158.0	150.0
7	11.0	118.3	132.3	129.4	112.9	135.1	120.7	178.0	212.0	160.0
8	8.5	132.2	140.0	106.6	119.1	142.1	92.9	170.6	180.0	104.7
9	11.0	127.7	137.8		108.5	137.6		186.4	278.2	
10	11.0	102.2	121.5			109.7	114.6		167.3	160.9
Mean ± SD	10.3 ± 1.6	119.8 ± 12.1	132.2 ± 6.7*	137.6 ± 22.1	115.0 ± 13.8	129.0 ± 11.9*	137.4 ± 34.9	185.3 ± 38.1	188.2 ± 47.6	161.9 ± 56.5

* $P < 0.02$ vs. prechallenge values

Source: from Takamura et al. (1997), p 146, table 1, with permission from Karger

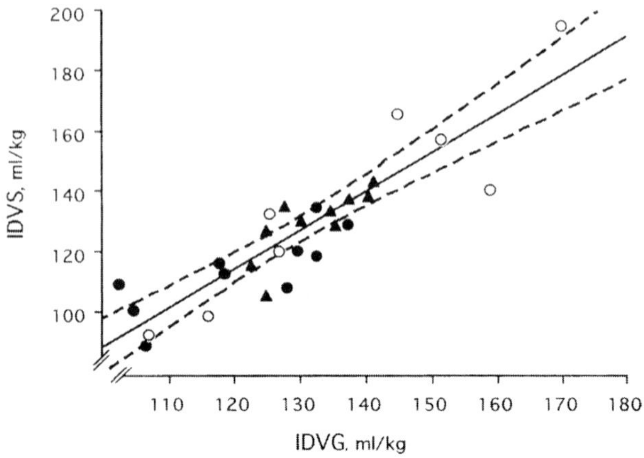

FIG. 5-2. Relationship between the initial distribution volume of glucose (*IDVG*) and the initial distribution volume of sucrose (*IDVS*) using a one-compartment model before the challenge (●), after the first challenge (▲), and after the second challenge (○). The *solid line* is a regression line obtained from all data: $Y = 1.28\ X - 39.1$ ($n = 28$, $r = 0.89$, $P < 0.0001$). *Dashed lines* indicate the 95% confidence interval for predicted IDVS for any given value of IDVG. (From Takamura et al. (1997), p 147, fig. 2, with permission from Karger)

Japan) was inserted into the left femoral artery to determine cardiac output (CO) and EVLW using a double indicator technique with chilled saline solution. The catheter was connected to the lung water computer (model MTV-1100; Nihon Kohden), which detects continuous changes in blood temperature and blood saline concentration in the femoral artery.

Before the first glucose administration, the CO and EVLW were measured using 5 ml chilled 5% saline solution; this served for the normovolemic or control values. Subsequently, both glucose 100 mg/kg and sucrose 100 mg/kg were infused simultaneously over 30 s through the femoral vein. Arterial blood samples were drawn to allow plasma glucose and sucrose concentrations to be measured immediately before and during 30 min postinfusion.

Ninety minutes after the end of blood sampling, blood was withdrawn at 1 ml/kg min over 30 min. Thirty minutes after completion of blood withdrawal, the second series of measurements and blood sampling were performed as before and served as the hypovolemic values. Ninety minutes after the end of the second series of blood sampling, 90 ml/kg lactated Ringer's solution was given over 30 min, followed by the third series of measurements and blood sampling to serve as the hypervolemic values.

TABLE 5-3. Changes in intial distribution volumes and extravascular lung water

	Normovolemia	Hypovolemia	Hypervolemia
IDVS ($ml\,kg^{-1}$)[a]	121.3 ± 22.1	85.7 ± 18.1*	137.9 ± 29.5**
Plasma sucrose (mg 100 ml^{-1})[b]	0	3.2 ± 2.8	6.1 ± 5.3**
IDVG ($ml\,kg^{-1}$)[c]	122.0 ± 20.8	96.0 ± 17.6*	145.3 ± 34.4*,**
Plasma glucose (mg 100 ml^{-1})[d]	109.6 ± 12.3	147.9 ± 44.3*	107.3 ± 29.9**
EVLW ($ml\,kg^{-1}$)	9.1 ± 2.7	7.9 ± 3.3	10.2 ± 3.1

IDVS, initial distribution volume of sucrose; IDVG, initial distribution volume of glucose; EVLW, extravascular lung water

Values are mean ± SD

[a] Akaike's information criterion (AIC) for plasma sucrose decay curve was –21.2 ± 5.8

[b] Plasma sucrose concentration present before sucrose infusion

[c] Akaike's information criterion (AIC) for plasma glucose decay curve was –22.5 ± 5.2

[d] Plasma glucose concentration present before glucose infusion

* $P < 0.05$ vs normovolemia; ** $P < 0.05$ vs hypovolemia

Source: from Iwakawa et al. (1998), p 416, table 1, with permission from Cambridge University Press

The mean IDVS during normovolemia was 121.3 ± 22.1 ml/kg, which decreased during hypovolemia ($P < 0.05$). The mean IDVS after volume loading increased, even though this was not statistically different from the normovolemic value (Table 5-3). The mean IDVG during normovolemia was 122.0 ± 20.8 ml/kg, which decreased with hypovolemia ($P < 0.05$) and subsequently increased with hypervolemia ($P < 0.05$). The mean EVLW during normovolemia was 9.1 ± 2.7 ml/kg. The value remained statistically unchanged throughout the procedure.

IDVG and IDVS individually changed together in the same direction following hypovolemia and subsequent hypervolemia in each dog. A good correlation was obtained between IDVG and IDVS ($r = 0.93$, $n = 36$, $P < 0.001$) (Fig. 5-3). When examining for an agreement between these two volumes using Bland and Altman's plots, the former was found to exceed the latter by an average of 6.1 ± 11.2 ml/kg (Fig. 5-4). A moderate correlation was obtained between IDVG and CO ($r = 0.75$, $n = 36$, $P < 0.001$). A poor correlation was found between IDVS and EVLW ($r = 0.38$, $n = 33$, $P < 0.05$) but not between IDVG and EVLW.

The mean urine volume during normovolemia was 4.4 ± 5.2 ml/kg over 90 min, followed by 1.6 ± 3.1 ml/kg over 90 min during hypovolemia, even though the difference was not statistically significant. The value increased to 22.9 ± 14.8 ml/kg over 90 min during hypervolemia compared with normovolemia ($P < 0.05$). We conclude that IDVG is a more useful indicator for the central ECF volume status than EVLW in a wide variety of fluid volume states.

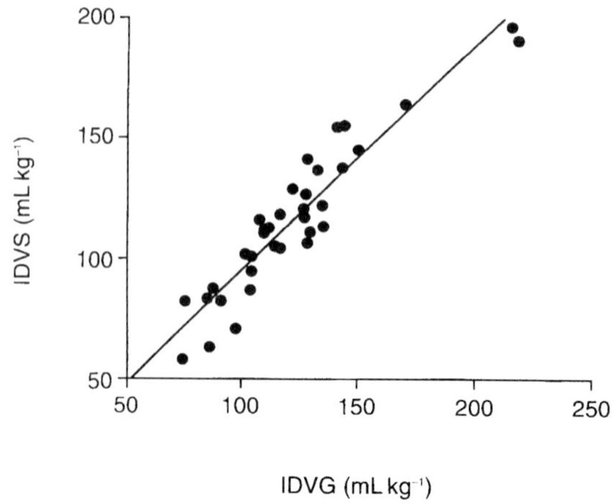

FIG. 5-3. Relationship between the initial distribution volume of glucose (*IDVG*) and the initial distribution volume of sucrose (*IDVS*) using a one-compartment model. *The straight line* is a regression line ($Y = 0.94X + 1.43$, $r = 0.93$, $P < 0.001$, $n = 36$). (From Iwakawa et al. (1998), p 417, fig. 1, with permission from Cambridge University Press)

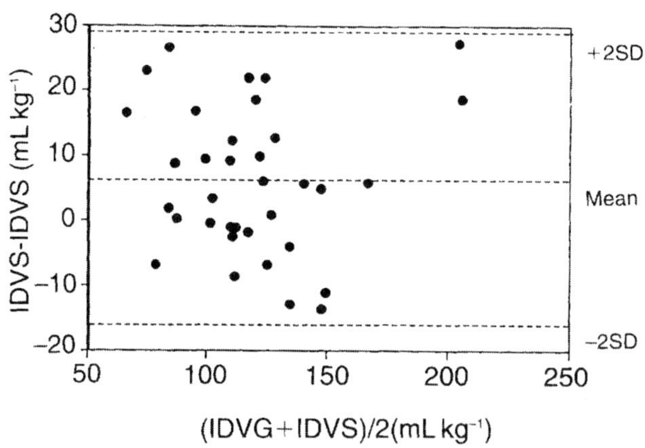

FIG. 5-4. Differences between the initial distribution volume of glucose (*IDVG*) and the initial distribution volume of sucrose (*IDVS*) versus their mean values according to Bland and Altman's method. *Dashed lines* represent mean and 95% confidence interval. (From Iwakawa et al. (1998), p 418, fig. 4, with permission from Cambridge University Press)

The Relationship Between IDVG and IDVS

These three studies consistently demonstrate a good linear correlation between IDVG and IDVS, and all dogs consistently showed that IDVG individually followed IDVS during the changes in the latter, indicating that IDVG represents the central extracellular fluid volume in a wide variety of fluid volume states. However, these two volumes are not equivalent, because sucrose has a larger molecular weight (342), nearly twice that of glucose (180), indicating that sucrose is less diffusible than glucose. Thus, IDVS would be slightly smaller than IDVG, as observed in these three studies. Additionally, there are some limitations of our studies.

First, sucrose administered previously was not completely cleared from the plasma at the time of repeated sucrose administration, which would modify the subsequent pharmacokinetic behavior of sucrose, because the reported elimination half-life of sucrose is relatively long: 71 ± 7 min (Bauer et al. 1990). However, residual plasma sucrose concentration before its administration was less than 10% of the corresponding plasma sucrose concentration at 3 min postadministration, and there was no correlation between the residual plasma sucrose concentration and IDVS during hypo- and subsequent hypervolemia in the third study. Second, in contrast to our previous fluid volume loading study by Miyahara et al. (1995) showing that each volume challenge increased both IDVG and plasma volume, the present fluid volume loading study described in this chapter failed to produce a consistent increase either in IDVG or IDVS. Urine volume between the second and the third administration of glucose and sucrose attained as much as the volume of the second fluid challenge (30 ml/kg), whereas urine volume measured in three dogs of the previous study using glucose and indocyanine green (ICG) as indicators (Miyahara et al. 1995) was less than 10 ml/kg during 60 min after each 30 ml/kg fluid volume challenge. This finding may be one reason why the fluid volume loading study described in this chapter failed to consistently induce a more-hypervolemic state, especially following the second volume challenge. The simultaneous administration of glucose and sucrose would yield a more hyperosmolar state in the plasma than that of glucose and ICG in the previous study (Miyahara et al. 1995). Five of eight dogs in this study had decreased CO following the second volume challenge. A relatively large blood sampling size throughout the experimental procedure (total, 120 ml) and a considerable amount of urine output may also be responsible for the decrease in CO.

A double indicator dilution technique, using a diffusible and a nondiffusible indicator, such as chilled ICG solution, has been used for measurement of EVLW (Schuster and Calandrino 1991). In the third experimental study described in this chapter, 5% chilled saline solution was used as the thermal diffusible and nondiffusible indicator previously reported (Ishibe and Suekane 1984). Its dilution curve reflects both the intravascular and extravascular compartments, as heat is dissipated across the endothelium into the surrounding lung tissue. Most of the injected saline stays in the intravascular compartment and provides an estimate of the intravascular compartment. A good agreement was obtained between the thermosaline method and the gravimetric measurement of lung water in experimental pulmonary edema (Ishibe and Suekane 1984). In addition, estimation of EVLW was thought to be accurate despite changes in CO over a wide range (Boldt et al. 1987). In the third study, there were no significant differences in the EVLW among different fluid volume states. Okumura et al. (1995) reported the effects of a fluid challenge on the EVLW in dogs. In their study, lactated Ringer's solution was infused at a rate of 90 ml/kgh for 30 min, and it was concluded that the pulmonary capillary permeability did not increase even after an excessive fluid challenge. Their result is comparable with that of the third study. Thus, the EVLW does not consistently indicate the generalized extravascular volume status of highly perfused organs, whereas IDVG may mirror it associated with the intravascular volume.

We employed a simultaneous glucose and sucrose administration in these three studies. However, this combination consistently produced an apparent hyperosmotic state that would itself modify fluid volume states. Therefore, the combination of these two indicators is not suitable for clinical purposes. However, IDVG was consistently correlated with IDVS in a wide variety of fluid volume states. The results of these three experimental studies indicate that IDVG can be used repeatedly as an indicator of the central ECF.

6. IDVG and Cardiac Output

The initial volume of distribution for several drugs is determined by cardiac output (CO), regional blood flow, and the characteristics of a particular drug (Ghoneim and Pearson 1990). After intravenous injection, drug concentrations in blood may be higher in individuals with poor perfusion (e.g., shock) than individuals with better perfusion (Bennet and Sheiner 1985). We have proposed that initial distribution volume of glucose (IDVG) mirrors the rapidly exchanging glucose pool as described in previous chapters. IDVG represents plasma volume and interstitial fluid volume of highly perfused tissues such as heart, lungs, brain, liver, and kidneys. Assuming that glucose metabolism does not have a significant impact on IDVG determination, IDVG may have a good correlation with CO. We found a linear correlation between these two variables in a patient after removal of pheochromocytoma in an early preliminary study (Ishihara et al. 1986a) (Fig. 6-1). Thereafter, we performed several experimental and clinical studies to examine the relationship between IDVG and CO in various pathological conditions.

Hemorrhagic Study

Twelve mongrel dogs weighing 7.0–9.0 kg were used for the experiments (Shimodate et al. 1994). Before glucose administration, CO was measured with 5 ml chilled normal saline solution. Then, 0.5 ml/kg glucose (100 mg/kg) was administered through the proximal port of the pulmonary artery catheter over 30 s. Blood samples were drawn immediately before and at 3, 5, and 7 min after the injection. Hemorrhage was induced by stepwise bleeding (1 ml/kg min) over 30 min. Thirty minutes after the completion of hemorrhage, a second series of measurements and blood sampling were performed. IDVG was calculated using a one-compartment model from the incremental plasma glucose decay curve between 3 and 7 min after glucose administration. Both IDVG and CO decreased after hemorrhage (Table 6-1). A

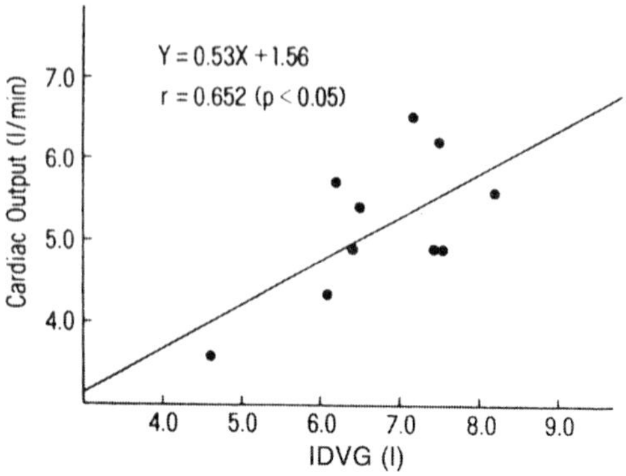

FIG. 6-1. Initial distribution volume of glucose (IDVG) and cardiac output in a surgical patient with pheochromocytoma. (From Ishihara et al. (1986a), p 77, fig. 2, with permission of Shinkokoueki)

TABLE 6-1. Initial distribution volume of glucose (IDVG) and cardiac output before and after hemorrhage

No.	BW (kg)	IDVG (l)		Cardiac output (l/min)	
		Before	After	Before	After
1	8.0	0.81	0.68	0.82	0.4
2	8.0	1.18	0.92	2.57	0.87
3	8.0	1.11	0.75	1.54	0.81
4	8.5	1.04	0.77	1.03	0.7
5	7.0	0.87	0.61	1.54	0.46
6	8.0	1.09	0.88	1.51	0.93
7	7.5	1.12	0.77	1.69	0.6
8	7.0	0.99	0.84	1.73	0.66
9	7.0	0.89	0.59	1.68	0.54
10	8.0	1.16	0.8	2.13	0.62
11	8.5	0.95	0.72	1.97	0.68
12	7.0	0.88	0.47	0.79	0.26
Mean ± SD	7.7 ± 0.6	1.01 ± 0.13	0.73 ± 0.13*	1.58 ± 0.52	0.63 ± 0.19*

BW, body weight; Before, before infusion; After, after infusion
* $P < 0.05$ versus before
Source: modified from Shimodate et al. (1994), p 259, table, with permission from the *Canadian Journal of Anesthesia*

correlation was found between IDVG and CO ($r = 0.85$, $n = 24$, $P < 0.001$). We conclude that IDVG correlates with CO following experimental hemorrhage.

Early Clinical Study in Critically Ill Patients

Thirteen nonsurgical patients who had a thermodilution pulmonary artery catheter were enrolled (Ishihara et al. 1993). Patients with congestive heart failure (CHF) judged from high pulmonary artery wedge pressure (>20 mmHg), echocardiography, or chest X-ray examination were excluded from the study. Ten patients were on vasoactive drugs, and 2 patients required continuous insulin infusions. A total of 27 comparisons between IDVG and thermodilution CO were performed. A bolus of 25 ml glucose 20% (5 g) was given over 30 s through the proximal port of a flow-directed pulmonary artery catheter. A glucose solution (5%–22%) for routine nutritional support was also infused through another central venous line using an electric pump at a constant rate, ranging from 0.1 to 0.4 g/kgh at least 1 h before the 5-g glucose challenge and throughout the procedure. Serial blood samples were obtained through an indwelling radial artery catheter immediately before and 3, 5, and 7 min after the glucose injection. IDVG was calculated in the same manner as described previously. CO was determined by triplicate measurements with 10 ml isotonic saline solution below 12°C injected in less than 4 s immediately after the completion of taking blood samples for glucose determination.

IDVG and CO varied markedly among the patients, ranging from 3.4 to 11.6 l for IDVG and from 3.4 to 14.0 l/min for CO, respectively. A linear correlation was obtained between IDVG and CO ($r = 0.89$, $n = 27$, $P < 0.001$) (Fig. 6-2). No correlation was found between IDVG and the preinjection plasma glucose concentration ($r = 0.007$). No difference was found between IDVG with or without continuous insulin or vasoactive drugs. We conclude that glucose metabolism has no apparent impact on determination of IDVG and that IDVG has a linear correlation with CO in the absence of CHF.

Clinical Study with or Without Congestive Heart Failure

In a previous clinical study, IDVG in critically ill patients without CHF was simply compared with CO. This study examined the relationship between these two variables with or without CHF. Forty-two patients having a flow-directed thermodilution pulmonary artery catheter, either surgical or nonsurgical, who were admitted to the general ICU were enrolled (Ishihara et al. 1996a). The patients were assigned to two groups according to the presence or absence of central extracellular fluid (ECF) volume accumulation. The

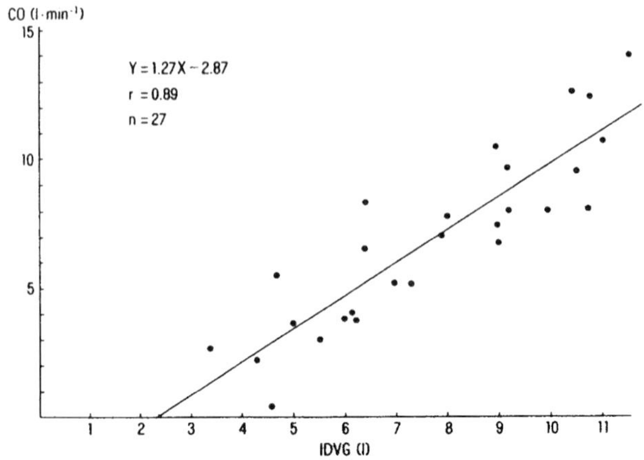

FIG. 6-2. Relationship between the initial distribution volume of glucose (IDVG) and cardiac output (CO). (From Ishihara et al. (1993), p 30, fig. 1, with permission from *Canadian Journal of Anesthesia*)

presence of the accumulation included CHF and/or obvious hypervolemia regardless of whether CO was maintained by vasoactive drugs. CHF was judged from the criteria described by McKee et al. (1971). Instead of increased central venous pressure, high pulmonary artery wedge pressure (>15 mmHg) was used. Seven patients met the criteria for diagnosis of the definite or probable CHF. Three patients with atrial fibrillation who also had persistent tachycardia (rate > 120/min) or ventricular premature contractions were considered to have relative fluid accumulation to their decreased CO, even though pulmonary artery wedge pressure was not increased. Four patients had apparent hypervolemia requiring ventilatory support, resulting from intravenous fluid overload as well as renal and/or cardiac dysfunction. Consequently, 14 patients met the criteria for diagnosis of the absolute or relative central ECF volume accumulation during their ICU stay. These patients served as the accumulation group. Comparison in each patient of IDVG to CO was conducted not more than four times on different days when physiological measurements and clinical signs showed the patient to be stable despite respiratory and/or cardiovascular support. A total of 81 comparisons were performed: 27 comparisons in the accumulation group and 54 in the nonaccumulation group. Vasoactive drugs such as norepinephrine were continuously infused during 36 comparisons. An insulin infusion was required during 19 comparisons. An infusion of 25 ml glucose 20% (5 g) was given over 30 s through the proximal port of the pulmonary artery catheter. Serial blood samples were obtained through an indwelling catheter placed in a radial artery immediately before and 3, 4, 5, and 7 min after the completion of glucose administration. IDVG was calculated from these values in the same manner as previously described.

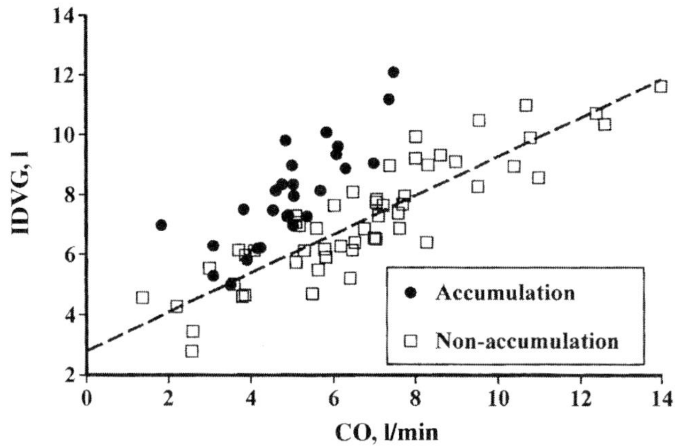

FIG. 6-3. Relationship between cardiac output (CO) and the initial distribution volume of glucose (IDVG) in critically ill patients with or without accumulation of the central extracellular fluid. *Dashed line* is a regression line obtained from data without accumulation: $Y = 0.6\,X + 2.8$ ($r = 0.89$, $n = 54$, $P < 0.001$). (From Ishihara et al. (1996a), *Infusionsther Transfusiosnmed* vol 23, p 199, fig. 1, with permission from Karger)

In the accumulation group, IDVG and CO varied markedly, ranging from 5.0 to 12.1 l for IDVG and from 1.8 to 7.4 l/min for CO. The highest CO value associated with the highest IDVG was obtained in a patient status postgastrojejunostomy with fluid overload requiring a large dose of norepinephrine infusion (1.0 µg/kg min) and continuous hemodiafiltration (CHDF) to treat renal dysfunction. In the nonaccumulation group, IDVG and CO also varied markedly, ranging from 2.8 to 11.7 l for IDVG and from 1.4 to 14.0 l/min for CO. The lowest CO was obtained in a severely burned patient with obvious hypovolemia during fluid resuscitation. A correlation was found between IDVG and CO ($r = 0.89$, $n = 54$, $P < 0.001$) (Fig. 6-3).

More than one comparison was conducted in 24 of 43 patients. Seven of these 24 patients (29%) failed to show IDVG and CO moving together toward the same direction. Results suggest that accumulation of the central ECF volume has a significant impact on the relationship between IDVG and CO in critically ill patients.

Clinical Study of IDVG and the Intravascular Volume After Esophagectomy

Thirty-one consecutive surgical patients admitted postoperatively to the general ICU were enrolled (Ishihara et al. 2000c). They underwent radical surgery for esophageal carcinoma, performed through a right thoracoabdominal approach with extensive resection of adjacent lymph nodes, subcarinal lymph nodes, and/or cervical lymph nodes, and stayed in the ICU for at least the first 3 postoperative days. Six patients received hemodilutional autologous blood transfusion, 4 patients received packed red blood cells, and 2 patients received colloidal solutions in the operating room.

A glucose-containing crystalloid solution was infused continuously for routine postoperative fluid management through a subclavian venous line using an electric pump at a constant rate: 1.4–2.2 ml/kgh for the first 2 days and 1.0–2.0 ml/kgh thereafter. However, lactated Ringer's solution (less than 2.0 l/day), colloidal solution (less than 0.75 l/day), and/or packed red blood cells (less than 2 units/day) were further administered as clinically required. Additionally, as part of their therapy, 4 patients during 13 measurements required an infusion of insulin, and 7 patients during 14 measurements required an infusion of vasoactive drugs such as dopamine, respectively. Diuretics such as furosemide were given in 6 patients on 8 different days. Patients required mechanical ventilatory support during their stay in the ICU for an average of 4.0 ± 2.4 days. Trachea remained intubated in 19 of 31 patients during the study period.

Postoperative IDVG and indocyanine green (ICG)-derived plasma volume (PV-ICG) were assessed immediately after admission to the ICU and daily between 9 and 10 A.M. for the first 3 postoperative days. Both 25 ml 20% glucose (5 g) and 10 ml ICG (25 mg) were infused simultaneously over 30 s through the proximal port of the pulmonary artery catheter. Continuous thermodilution CO (Vigilance Monitor, model VGSSYS; Baxter Healthcare, Irvine, CA, USA) and other routine clinical variables were recorded immediately before each measurement of these two volumes. Body weight was measured immediately after admission to the ICU and subsequently each day at 8:30 A.M.

Serial blood samples were obtained through an indwelling radial or femoral artery catheter at the following times: immediately before and 1, 2, 3, 4, 5, 7, 9, and 11 min after the completion of both ICG and glucose infusions. PV-ICG was calculated utilizing a one-compartment model from the plasma ICG concentrations from 3 to 9 or 11 min postinfusion in the same manner as described in Chapter 7. Circulating blood volume was then calculated by utilizing PV-ICG and hematocrit (BV-ICG). Fluid volumes in this study have been adjusted to a single bolus injection using a mathematical equation proposed by Loo and Riegelman (1970), as described in Chapter 1.

Median values of increased body weight above the preoperative value, administered crystalloid solutions, and urine output after surgery on the operative day were 2.0 kg, 2.2 ml/kgh, and 0.6 ml/kgh, respectively. Although an increase in body weight remained even on the third postoperative day, the amounts of administered crystalloid solutions decreased, and there was an associated increase in urine output ($P < 0.05$). Hematocrit decreased on the second and third postoperative days compared to the operative day ($P < 0.05$). In addition, total plasma protein concentrations decreased on the third postoperative day ($P < 0.05$).

Median values of IDVG, PV-ICG, BV-ICG, and cardiac index (CI) after surgery on the operative day were 3.5 l/m^2, 1.6 l/m^2, 2.4 l/m^2, and 3.2 l/min m^2, respectively (Table 6-2). IDVG and PV-ICG increased along with CI on the second and the third postoperative days when compared with the operative day ($P < 0.05$). However, a statistically significant increase in BV-ICG was observed only on the third postoperative day ($P < 0.05$). Red cell volume obtained by subtracting PV-ICG from the corresponding BV-ICG decreased on the second and the third postoperative days compared to the operative day ($P < 0.05$). Although mean arterial pressure (MAP) decreased on the second and the third postoperative days compared with the operative day ($P < 0.05$), pulmonary artery wedge pressure and central venous pressure (CVP) remained at less than 16 mmHg and remained unchanged throughout the study period.

IDVG had a better correlation with CI when compared with either PV-ICG or BV-ICG ($r = 0.71$ for IDVG, $r = 0.45$ for PV-ICG, and $r = 0.23$ for BV-ICG) (Fig. 6-4). No correlation was also found between MAP and CI ($r = -0.14$), pulmonary artery wedge pressure, and CI ($r = 0.04$) or CVP and CI ($r = -0.08$). We conclude that IDVG rather than the intravascular volume has a better correlation with CO after major surgical procedures.

TABLE 6-2. Cardiovascular and fluid volume values (median, range) in the first postoperative days

	Day 0	Day 1	Day 2	Day 3
CI (l min^{-1} m^{-2})	3.2 (1.8–5.4)	2.9 (1.5–4.2)	3.5 (2.2–5.4)	4.0 (2.8–6.9)*
MAP (mmHg)	93 (66–121)	84 (57–108)	82 (53–113)*	79 (55–119)*
PAWP (mmHg)	8 (4–14)	7 (4–13)	8 (2–16)	8 (2–15)
CVP (mmHg)	7 (−1–14)	6 (0–15)	6 (1–10)	7 (2–13)
IDVG (l m^{-2})	3.5 (2.7–5.1)	3.5 (2.7–4.8)	3.9 (2.6–5.6)*	4.3 (3.3–5.6)*
PV-ICG (l m^{-2})	1.6 (1.1–2.0)	1.4 (1.2–2.3)	1.6 (1.0–2.6)*	1.8 (1.4–2.4)*
BV-ICG (l m^{-2})	2.4 (1.7–2.9)	2.2 (1.6–3.7)	2.2 (1.5–3.7)	2.5 (1.9–3.2)*
RCV (l m^{-2})	0.8 (0.4–1.3)	0.7 (0.4–1.4)	0.7 (0.5–1.1)*	0.6 (0.4–1.0)*

CI, cardiac index; MAP, mean arterial pressure; PAWP, pulmonary artery wedge pressure; CVP, central venous pressure; IDVG, initial distribution volume of glucose; PV-ICG, plasma volume determined using indocyanine dilution; BV-ICG, blood volume derived from PV-ICG and hematocrit; RCV, red blood cell volume derived from BV-ICG and PV-ICG

* $P < 0.05$ vs day 0

Source: from Ishihara et al. (2000c), p 1444, table 3, with permission from Springer

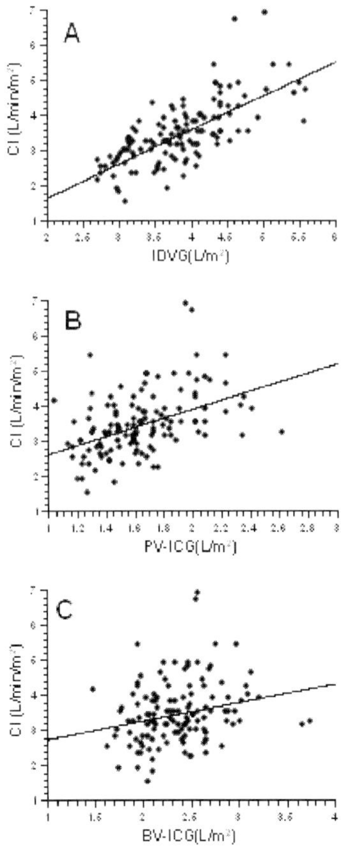

FIG. 6-4. Relationship during the first postoperative days following radical surgery for esophageal carcinoma cardiac index (*CI*) and initial distribution volume of glucose (*IDVG*, **A**), plasma volume determined by the ICG dilution method (*PV-ICG*, **B**), and blood volume determined by PV-ICG and hematocrit (*BV-ICG*, **C**). **A** IDVG vs CI: $Y = 0.97X - 0.29$, $r = 0.71$, $n = 124$, $P < 0.000001$; **B** PV-ICG vs CI: $Y = 1.29X + 1.34$, $r = 0.45$, $n = 124$, $P < 0.000001$; **C** BV-ICG vs CI: $Y = 0.53X + 2.2$, $r = 0.23$, $n = 124$, $P < 0.01$. (From Ishihara et al. (2000c), p 1445, fig. 2, with permission from Springer)

Relationship Between IDVG and Cardiac Output

Results consistently demonstrated that IDVG had a good linear correlation with CO in the experimental hemorrhagic study as well as in clinical studies in the absence of CHF, even though our early studies had study design limitations, such as a different sampling size from each patient and only three points being used for calculation of IDVG. However, IDVG was poorly correlated with CO in our two experimental studies: fluid volume loading (Miyahara et al. 1995) (Fig. 6-5) and phentolamine infusion (Matsui et al. 2000). These results are contrast to our previous assumption based on pharmacokinetic behavior of initial distribution volume consistently reflecting CO (Ghoneim and Pearson 1990). In contrast, IDVG itself may have an obvious impact on determination of CO similar to cardiac preload, even though intravenously administered glucose does not stay in the intravascular compartment, even soon after administration. As CO depends on cardiac

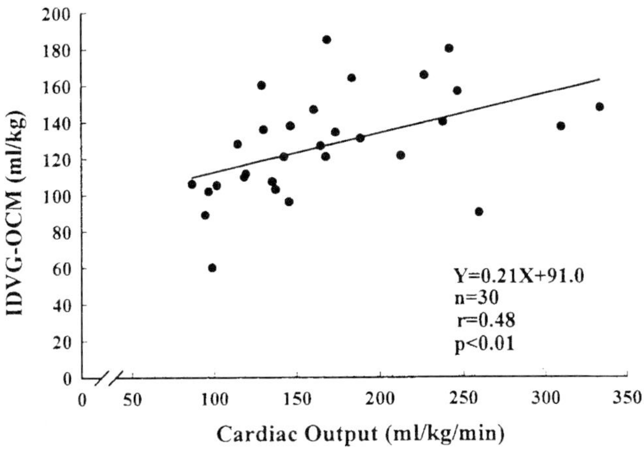

FIG. 6-5. Relationship between IDVG using a one-compartment model (IDVG-OCM) and cardiac output by the thermodilution method (CO). (From Miyahara et al. (1995), p 277, fig. 3, with permission from Karger)

preload based on the Frank–Starling relationship, the better the filling of the heart, the better the forward output. This relationship was observed in our study, in which IDVG had a good correlation with CO. In our experimental fluid volume challenge study, however, the left ventricle would have reached near maximal size by the first volume challenge (30 ml/kg). Accordingly, subsequent volume challenge (30 ml/kg) would fail to induce a further increase in end-diastolic diameter. Furthermore, the largest fluid volume challenge (60 ml/kg) induced a decrease in CO despite an increase in IDVG in one of three dogs (Table 6-3). Additionally, CO and IDVG did not move together toward the same direction in nearly one-third of critically ill patients who had more than two IDVG and CO measurements (Ishihara et al. 1996a). The same study also demonstrated that IDVG in the presence of either CHF or fluid overload is larger than that in its absence. These findings suggest that IDVG would not be correlated with CO when cardiac preload is on the descending part of the Frank–Starling curve. Myocardial contractility, cardiac afterload, and heart rate also play a role in determining CO as observed during phentolamine infusion (Matsui et al. 2000). The contribution of cardiac preload and afterload on either IDVG or CO is discussed in Chapter 9.

Based on capillary membrane permeability of glucose, the rate at which glucose molecules diffuse through the capillary membrane is approximately 50 times greater than the rate at which plasma itself flows linearly along the capillary (Guyton and Hall 2000a). Presumably, CO itself has a minimal

TABLE 6-3. IDVG, plasma volume, and cardiac output preinfusion (pre-inf.) and postinfusion (post-inf.) (60 ml/kg 3% dextran in lactated Ringer's solution)

No.	BW (kg)	IDVG (ml/kg)		Plasma volume (ml/kg)		Cardiac output (ml/kg min)	
		pre-inf.	post-inf.	pre-inf.	post-inf.	pre-inf.	post-inf.
1	11.0	90.9	115.5	45.5	84.5	176	226
2	11.0	100.0	137.3	56.4	79.1	185	125
3	10.0	113.0	147.0	59.0	86.0	188	258
Mean	10.7	101.3	133.3	53.6	83.2	183	203

BW, body weight
Source: from Miyahara et al. (1995), p 278, table 2, with permission from Karger

effect on glucose distribution, and thus IDVG determination whether CO is decreased. Therefore, measurement of IDVG is reliable even in a state of low CO.

We have proposed that the IDVG/CO ratio is useful as an index of fluid accumulation in the central compartment (Ishihara et al. 1996a). The ratio of presence or the absence of CHF was 1.68 ± 0.47 and 1.16 ± 0.40, respectively. The higher the IDVG/CO ratio, the greater the deterioration in cardiac function and/or the greater accumulation of fluid in the central compartment of each individual patient. The combined data in clinical study on postesophagectomy yielded a IDVG/CO ratio of 1.16 ± 0.22, indicating that neither apparent cardiac dysfunction nor central fluid accumulation is likely even in a relatively low CO state observed during the first 3 postoperative days (Ishihara et al. 2000c). Thus, central hypovolemia requiring subsequent fluid volume loading would play a key role in developing relatively low CO in the early postoperative period following esophagectomy, although neither mean arterial pressure, pulmonary artery wedge pressure, nor CVP consistently identified its presence.

We also demonstrated that IDVG rather than the intravascular volume including plasma volume and blood volume is correlated with CO following esophagectomy or even early after percutaneous coronary angioplasty in acute myocardial infarction patients (Ishihara et al. 2000d), suggesting that IDVG rather than the intravascular volume has the potential of being an alternative measure of cardiac preload. Additionally, plasma or blood volume does not consistently have a significant impact on determination of CO. Fluid redistribution between the central and peripheral tissues may affect cardiac preload, even if the intravascular volume state remains unchanged as observed in our experimental study following phentolamine infusion (Matsui et al. 2000).

7. IDVG and Plasma Volume

In Chapter 5, we showed a good correlation of the initial distribution volume of glucose (IDVG) with the central extracellular fluid (ECF) volume in a wide variety of fluid volume states. In this chapter, IDVG is compared with plasma volume derived by the indocyanine green (ICG) dilution method (Vd-ICG or PV-ICG) (Koh et al. 1995; Miyahara et al. 1995). Additionally, we discuss some issues of ICG-derived distribution volume.

ICG as an Indicator of Plasma Volume Measurement

ICG is a water-soluble tricarbocyanine dye that contains 5.0%–9.5% sodium iodide. Adverse reactions to this dye are very rare, but life-threatening anaphylactic reaction can occur (Benya et al. 1989). When injected into the bloodstream, ICG rapidly binds to plasma proteins (Hwang et al. 1975) and is distributed throughout the circulating intravascular compartment. ICG is taken up by hepatic parenchymal cells and is excreted unchanged into the bile. ICG has been used for estimating plasma volume (Henschen et al. 1993) and circulating blood volume calculated from PV-ICG and hematocrit values (He et al. 1998). Its accuracy is equal to the radioisotopic method utilizing ^{51}Cr-labeled red cells (Busse et al. 1993). As the peak absorption for ICG is 805 nm, its determinations can be performed simply by a spectrophotometric assay. Additionally, as this dye has a short half-life, around 3 min for healthy humans, repeated measurements can be performed at a 30-min interval when hepatic function is normal (Haruna et al. 1998). In contrast, more than 30% of the administered ICG remains in the intravascular compartment even at 60 min postinjection when hepatic function is extremely impaired (disappearance rate of ICG from plasma, less than 0.02/min). Accuracy of the repeated measurement can be confirmed by comparing red cell volume

(RCV) derived by PV-ICG and hematocrit in each measurement when apparent internal or external bleeding is negligible.

Although accurate physiological assessment of the pharmacokinetic behavior of ICG requires at least a two-compartment model (TCM) (Avram et al. 1990; Sekimoto et al. 1997), the ICG dilution method for plasma volume measurement or hepatic blood flow has been traditionally performed by fitting a one-compartment model (OCM) to plasma ICG concentration versus time data (Haller et al. 1993; Busse et al. 1993). When examining for the agreement of PV-ICG between an OCM and a TCM in 12 patients using the statistical method described by Bland and Altman (Ishihara et al. 1999), the former was found to exceed the latter by an average of 0.07 ± 0.08 l. Therefore, the 95% confidence limits for agreement between two volumes were from −0.36 to 0.23 l. Consequently, an OCM is clinically acceptable for plasma volume measurement.

Hemorrhagic Study

Eight dogs weighing 6.0–10.3 kg were used for the experiments (Koh et al. 1995). All dogs were intubated and mechanically ventilated under pentobarbital anesthesia. Both 0.1 g/kg glucose and 0.5 mg/kg ICG were infused simultaneously through the proximal port of the pulmonary artery catheter over 30 s. Blood samples were drawn immediately before and at 3, 5, 7, and 9 min after the injection, respectively. Two hours after the infusion, hemorrhage was induced by stepwise bleeding (1 ml/kg min) over 30 min. Thirty minutes after completion of the hemorrhage, a second series of glucose and ICG infusions and blood sampling were repeated as before the hemorrhage.

Plasma glucose concentrations were measured using the glucose oxidase method. Plasma ICG concentrations were measured using a spectrophotometric technique (U3200 spectrophotometer; Hitachi, Tokyo, Japan). IDVG and Vd-ICG were calculated using an OCM: incremental plasma concentrations were between 3 and 7 min postinjection for IDVG and between 3 and 9 min for Vd-ICG, respectively.

The mean IDVG was 114 ± 13 ml/kg before hemorrhage, which decreased to 87 ± 15 ml/kg after hemorrhage (Table 7-1). The mean Vd-ICG was reduced from 50 ± 6 ml/kg to 35 ± 6 ml/kg. A linear correlation was obtained between IDVG and Vd-ICG ($r = 0.85$, $n = 16$, $P < 0.001$) (Fig. 7-1). We conclude that IDVG correlates with Vd-ICG following experimental hemorrhage.

TABLE 7-1. Initial distribution volume of glucose (IDVG) and indocyanine green-derived plasma volume (Vd-ICG) before and after hemorrhage

No.	BW (kg)	IDVG ($ml\,kg^{-1}$)		Vd-ICG ($ml\,kg^{-1}$)	
		B	A	B	A
1	7.5	130	65	47	28
2	7.5	104	93	49	40
3	7.7	120	82	53	35
4	8.5	101	81	44	30
5	10.1	111	99	53	36
6	8.5	127	74	43	27
7	6.0	123	114	61	46
8	10.3	97	88	49	36
	8.3 ± 1.4	114 ± 13	87 ± 15*	50 ± 6	35 ± 6†

Values are mean ± SD

B, before hemorrhage; A, after hemorrhage; IDVG, initial distribution volume of glucose; Vd-ICG, ICG dilution assessments of plasma volume

* $P < 0.02$ versus B; † $P < 0.001$ versus B

Source: from Koh et al. (1995), p 165, table, with permission from *Canadian Journal of Anesthesia*

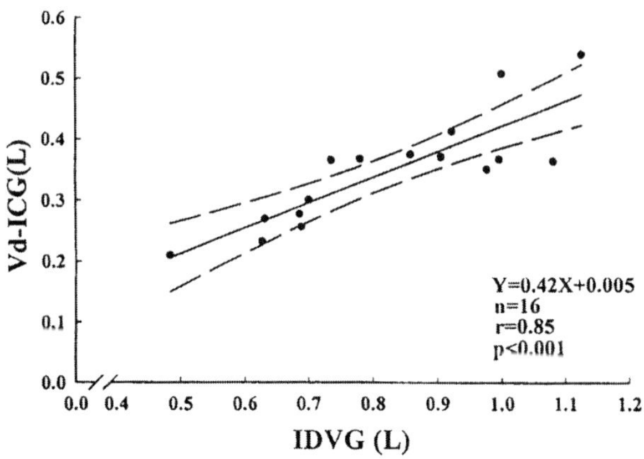

FIG. 7-1. Relationship between the initial distribution volume of glucose (IDVG) using a one-compartment model and the distribution volume of indocyanine green (Vd-ICG) in normovolemic and hypovolemic dogs. *Solid line* is a regression line obtained from all data: $Y = 0.42X + 0.005$ ($r = 0.85$, $n = 16$, $P < 0.001$); *dashed lines* indicate 95% confidence interval for predicted Vd-ICG for any given values of IDVG. (From Koh et al. (1995), p 165, fig. 1, with permission from *Canadian Journal of Anesthesia*)

Fluid Volume Loading Study

Thirteen mongrel dogs of either sex weighing 9.0–14.5 kg were used (Miyahara et al. 1995). Preparatory procedures were essentially the same as the hemorrhagic study already described. Before the glucose administration, cardiac output (CO) was measured with 5 ml chilled lactated Ringer's solution. Subsequently, both glucose 0.1 g/kg and ICG 0.5 mg/kg were administered simultaneously through the proximal port of the pulmonary artery catheter over 30 s. Blood samples were drawn immediately before and at 3, 4, 5, 7, 9, 11, 15, 25, and 30 min. Then, 30 ml/kg 3% dextran in lactate Ringer's solution was given twice over 30 min at an interval of 2.5 h. Repeated measurements and blood samplings were performed at 30 min after each completion of infusion in the same manner as performed before the volume challenge.

IDVG was calculated using an OCM from the incremental plasma glucose decay curve between 3 and 7 min after glucose administration. PV-ICG was calculated using an OCM from the incremental plasma ICG decay curve between 3 and 9 min after ICG administration.

The mean preinfusion IDVG was 112.8 ± 28.7 ml/kg, which increased after the first and second fluid volume infusions ($P < 0.05$) (Table 7-2). The mean preinfusion PV-ICG was 59.5 ± 12.3 ml/kg, which increased after the first and second fluid volume infusions ($P < 0.05$). A linear correlation was obtained between IDVG and PV-ICG ($r = 0.79$, $n = 30$, $P < 0.001$) (Fig. 7-2). We conclude that IDVG correlates with PV-ICG following experimental fluid volume challenge.

TABLE 7-2. Cardiovascular variables and IDVG following volume challenge

	Preinfusion	First infusion	Second infusion
Cardiac output (ml/kg min)	157 ± 53	174 ± 69	178 ± 64
Heart rate (beats/min)	162 ± 29	138 ± 34*	133 ± 40*
Mean arterial pressure (mmHg)	131 ± 20	136 ± 16*	137 ± 19*
Pulmonary artery wedge pressure (mmHg)	9.1 ± 4.0	12.6 ± 5.2*	12.1 ± 2.3*
Central venous pressure (mmHg)	7.9 ± 2.3	8.4 ± 1.7*	10.2 ± 3.0*
PV-ICG (ml/kg)	59.5 ± 12.3	75.9 ± 16.1*	81.1 ± 16.9*
IDVG (ml/kg)	112.8 ± 28.7	133.6 ± 27.7*	135.7 ± 21.5*

Values are mean ± SD

* $P < 0.05$ compared with preinfusion

Source: modified from Miyahara et al. (1995), p 276, table 1, with permission from Karger

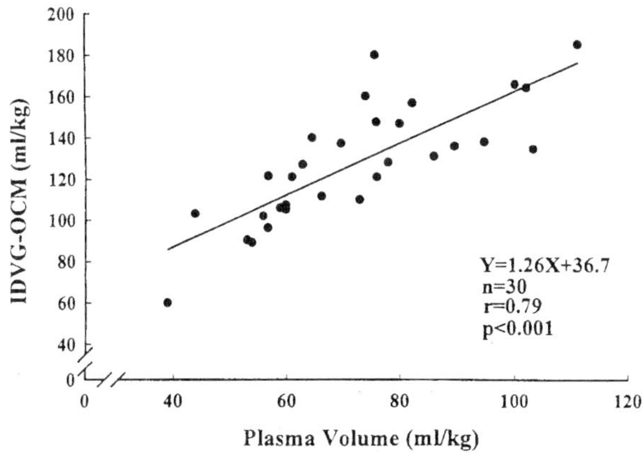

FIG. 7-2. Relationship between IDVG using a one-compartment model (IDVG-OCM) and plasma volume by the ICG dilution method. (from Miyahara et al. (1995), p 277, fig. 2, with permission from Karger)

Accuracy of ICG-Derived Plasma Volume (PV-ICG)

The most important inaccuracy of PV-ICG measurement would be overestimation of PV-ICG when apparent general protein capillary leakage is present, which is described in Chapter 8. Additionally, as this dye is exclusively excreted from the liver, its reduced excretion may affect not only the disappearance rate of ICG from plasma (Ke-ICG), but also PV-ICG, because accuracy of the compartment model is based only on the normal physiological state. Assuming that PV-ICG can be measured accurately regardless of the magnitude of Ke-ICG, convergence should be assumed in each ICG clearance curve. In addition, a close linear correlation should be obtained between PV-ICG and a reliable method of plasma volume determination, such as a radioisotopic method utilizing ^{51}Cr-labeled red cells (Busse et al. 1993).

Although IDVG is not proportionally greater than plasma volume, the mean PV-ICG/IDVG ratio remained unchanged regardless of hemorrhage (30 ml/kg) or volume challenge (30 ml/kg) when the ratio was calculated using data from the two experimental studies described previously (Koh et al. 1995; Miyahara et al. 1995). Considering pharmacokinetic behavior of glucose, no direct measurements of accuracy of PV-ICG in each patient could be performed using IDVG as a reference. However, assuming that the relationship between these two volumes remained unchanged regardless of the magnitude of the Ke-ICG, ICG would accurately measure plasma volume independently of the Ke-ICG, as ICG has been reported to measure plasma volume accurately when the Ke-ICG is normal (Henschen et al. 1993; Iijima et al. 1998).

A total of 193 consecutive adult patients, either postsurgical or medical, admitted to the general intensive care unit (ICU) were initially enrolled (Ishihara et al. 1999). Twenty-one patients among the 193 patients had a PV-ICG/IDVG ratio greater than 0.45 and were also excluded from the study because of possible overestimation of the PV-ICG, which is described in more detail in the next chapter. The remaining 172 patients were allocated retrospectively to one of the following four groups according to the magnitude of the Ke-ICG: the low group (Ke-ICG <0.10, $n = 40$), the 10 group ($0.1 \leqq$ Ke-ICG < 0.2, $n = 52$), the 20 group ($0.2 \leqq$ Ke-ICG < 0.3, $n = 55$), and the high group (Ke-ICG $\geqq 0.30$, $n = 24$) (Table 7-3). The data of the first determination of each patient only were used for the study. As part of their therapy, 100 patients required mechanical ventilation, 54 patients required an infusion of insulin, and 95 patients required an infusion of vasoactive drugs such as adrenaline, noradrenaline, dobutamine, and dopamine.

Both 25 ml glucose 20% (5 g) and 10 ml ICG (25 mg) were infused simultaneously over 30 s through the central venous catheter. IDVG and PV-ICG were calculated utilizing an OCM from the increased plasma value between 3 and 7 min postinfusion for the former and between 3 to 9 or 11 min postinfusion for the latter.

Although body weight and plasma glucose concentrations present before glucose challenge were not different among groups (see Table 7-3 and Table 7-4), the age of the low group was greater than that of the high group ($P <$ 0.05). Both the APACHE II score (Knaus et al. 1985) and the total bilirubin concentration in blood were higher in the low group than in the other groups ($P < 0.05$ and $P < 0.001$, respectively). A considerable number of patients died during their stay in the ICU, except in the high group. The median Akaike's information criterion (AIC) value of the ICG clearance curve was –41.4 (range, –65.7 to –32.3) for the low group and was not different among the other groups. The median AIC value of the glucose clearance curve was –23.5 (–34.2 to –17.6) for the low group and was not different among the other groups. The lowest Ke-ICG in the low group was 0.016/min, associated with the AIC value of –39.1 for this ICG curve. The highest Ke-ICG of the high group was 0.428/min associated with the AIC value of –33.1. As judged from the AIC values, convergence was consistently assumed in either the ICG or the glucose clearance curve, even in the low Ke-ICG.

Hematocrit in the low group was significantly lower than that of the 10 group ($P < 0.05$) and the high group ($P < 0.05$) (Table 7-4). Both IDVG and PV-ICG in the low group was significantly larger than in the 10 group ($P < 0.05$). These data indicated the presence of fluid accumulation in the low group. However, the PV-ICG/IDVG ratio was 0.38 for the low group, and no statistically significant difference was observed among groups. A linear correlation was obtained between IDVG and PV-ICG in the low group ($r = 0.84$,

TABLE 7-3. Patient profile of each group

Group	Low (Ke-ICG < 0.1)	10 (0.1 ≦ Ke-ICG < 0.2)	20 (0.2 ≦ Ke-ICG < 0.3)	High (0.3 ≦ Ke-ICG)
Number of patients	40	52	55	24
Age (years)	68 (28–85)	67.5 (26–87)	64 (28–83)	58 (21–72)*
BW (kg)	60.1 (39.8–98.2)	58.0 (41.8–92.3)	60.0 (39.9–90.5)	63.9 (45.4–91.5)
Medical/postoperative patients	18/22	18/34	12/43	15/9
APACHE II score	17 (4–33)	11 (0–28)*	11 (1-23)*	8.5 (2–27)*
Bilirubin (mg/100 ml)	3.4 (0.5–21.6)	1.0 (0.3–6.6)**	0.8 (0.2–12.2)**	0.75 (0.2–2.3)**
Nonsurvivor	13	7	8	0
Ventilatory support	27	30	25	18
Insulin	12	18	14	10
Vasoactive drugs	22	36	29	8

Values are median (range)

Ke-ICG, disappearance rate of indocyanine green (ICG) from plasma; BW, reported basal body weight; APACHE, Acute Physiology and Chronic Health Evaluation; bilirubin, total bilirubin concentration in blood; nonsurvivor, number of patients who died during their stay in the ICU; ventilatory support, number of patients requiring mechanical ventilatory support; insulin, number of patients receiving a continuous insulin infusion; vasoactive drugs, number of patients receiving a continuous infusion of vasoactive drugs, i.e., dopamine, dobutamine, noradrenaline, and adrenaline

* $P < 0.05$ versus the low groups; ** $P < 0.001$ versus the low group

Source: from Ishihara et al. (1999), p 1254, table 1, with permission from Springer

TABLE 7-4. Pharmacokinetic variables

Group	Low (Ke-ICG < 0.1)	10 (0.1 ≦ Ke-ICG < 0.2)	20 (0.2 ≦ Ke-ICG < 0.3)	High (0.3 ≦ Ke-ICG)
Plasma glucose (mmol/l)	8.0 (4.2–16.0)	8.7 (5.1–16.1)	8.1 (4.5–15.9)	8.7 (3.1–11.6)
IDVG (l)	7.30 (3.84–12.22)	6.31 (4.23–9.44)*	6.58 (4.92–10.30)	6.78 (4.60–10.34)
Ke-glucose (/min)	0.06 (0.03–0.17)	0.07 (0.04–0.11)	0.07 (0.03–0.11)	0.08 (0.06–0.14)*
PV-ICG (L)	2.64 (1.51–4.77)	2.34 (1.54–3.38)*	2.38 (1.53–3.99)	2.46 (1.66–3.58)
PV-ICG/IDVG ratio	0.38 (0.25–0.44)	0.38 (0.28–0.44)	0.36 (0.27–0.44)	0.35 (0.29–0.43)
Hematocrit (%)	29.1 (14.2–42.2)	34.0 (22.2–56.5)*	31.6 (16.4–59.3)	34.3 (12.7–53.0)*

Values are median (range)

Ke-ICG, disappearance rate of indocyanine green; (ICG), from plasma; plasma glucose concentration present immediately before glucose administration; IDVG, initial distribution volume of glucose; Ke-glucose, disappearance rate of glucose from plasma; PV-ICG, plasma volume determined by the ICG dilution method

* $P <$ versus the low group

Source: from Ishihara et al. (1999), p 1255, table 2, with permission from Springer

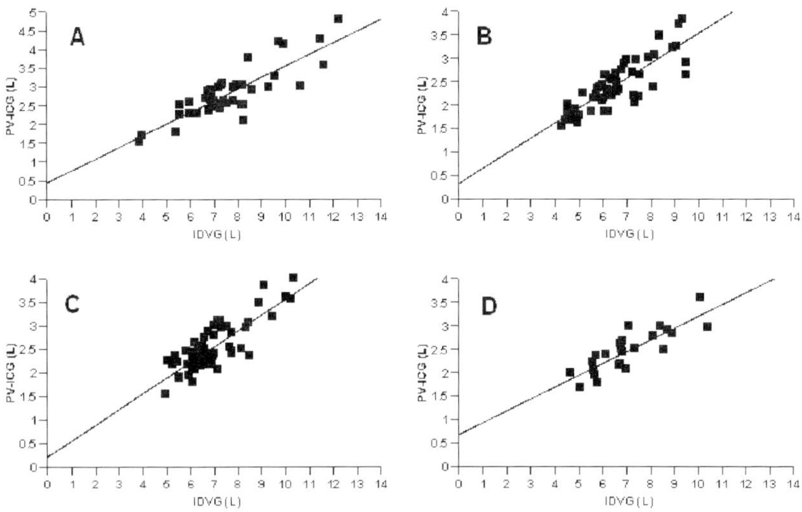

FIG. 7-3A–D. Relationship between initial distribution volume of glucose (*IDVG*) and plasma volume (*PV-ICG*) determined by the indocyanine green (*ICG*) dilution method. **A** Low group: $Y = 0.3X + 0.4$, $r = 0.84$, $n = 40$, $P < 0.001$; **B** 10 group: $Y = 0.3X + 0.3$, $r = 0.82$, $n = 52$, $P < 0.001$; **C** 20 group: $Y = 0.3X + 0.2$, $r = 0.82$, $n = 55$, $P < 0.001$; **D** high group: $Y = 0.2X + 0.6$, $r = 0.83$, $n = 24$, $P < 0.001$. (From Ishihara et al. (1999), p 1255, fig. 1, with permission from Springer)

$n = 40$, $P < 0.001$). The relationship between the two volumes was not different among groups (Fig. 7-3).

These findings would suggest that the relationship between the two volumes remains unchanged even during fluid accumulation associated with a low Ke-ICG. The PV-ICG/IDVG ratio in this study varied considerably among patients, ranging between 0.25 and 0.44, as observed in our previous studies (Ishihara et al. 1998c, 2000d). We believe that this considerable variability reflects the intra- and extravascular volume status in each patient and is not caused by the methodological flaws of IDVG determination.

Although a statistical difference was not observed in the PV-ICG/IDVG ratio among groups, the relationship between the two volumes in the high group seems to be different from other groups, as indicated by a relatively low median PV-ICG/IDVG ratio in the high group compared to the other groups. Schroder et al. (1999) reported that the higher the Ke-ICG, the greater the error of PV-ICG would occur, as recirculation of ICG within 60 s postinjection significantly affects its pharmacokinetic behavior. An increase in the disappearance rate of glucose from plasma (Ke-glucose) was also observed in the high group, suggesting that glucose in the central compartment moves rapidly into the peripheral compartment by insulin-like activity or some unknown mechanism independent of its distribution volume in this group. This phenomenon is caused by increased exchange between plasma and interstitial fluid and is not related to glucose transport into the cells (Chinkes et al. 1995). Presumably, glucose metabolism does not obviously affect measurement of IDVG, even in the high group.

Given that the reported normal Ke-ICG is 0.156 ± 0.064/min (Ishigami et al. 1993), a wide variety of Ke-ICG was observed in this study. Results also suggest that critically ill patients are likely to have hepatic dysfunction, as reported previously (Maynard et al. 1997), because a considerable number of patients in this study had a low Ke-ICG associated with a high total bilirubin concentration in blood, even though these variables did not consistently indicate hepatic dysfunction. Twelve patients of the low group (30%) had Ke-ICG less than 0.06/min, indicating poor outcome according to a previous report (Kholoussy et al. 1984). In fact, 9 of these 12 patients (75%) died during their stay in the ICU. A higher APACHE II score (Knaus et al. 1985) in the low group compared to other groups would also support the presence of the life-threatening underlying pathological state in the low group.

Eighteen patients among 60 patients in whom thermodilution CO was measured simultaneously with the two distribution volumes had a low cardiac output (less than 2.5 l/min m^2). When examining for agreement between PV-ICG utilizing data beginning at 3 min postinfusion and that at 5 min postinfusion using the statistical method described by Bland and Altman, the former was found to underestimate the latter by an average of 0.06 l. The standard deviation of the difference between two volumes was 0.09 l. Therefore, the 95% confidence limits for agreement between two volumes were from −0.24 to 0.12 l. Although Sekimoto et al. (1997) recommended using data beginning at 5 min or thereafter to calculate PV-ICG in low CO states, underestimation of PV-ICG using data beginning at 3 min postinfusion would be clinically negligible, judged by the result of the Bland and Altman method. We conclude that measurement of PV-ICG can be equally accurate independently of its disappearance rate from plasma unless there is generalized protein capillary leakage.

Relationship Between IDVG and Plasma Volume

In our experimental and clinical studies, data from 3 to 9 or 11 min postinfusion were fitted to an OCM, as conducted similarly in other studies (Henthorn et al. 1989; Haruna et al. 1998). Based on results of our simultaneous measurements of IDVG and PV-ICG, IDVG has approximately 2–2.5 times greater volume than PV-ICG, unless there is no apparent overestimation of PV-ICG. However, IDVG should not be used as a surrogate measure of plasma volume because IDVG is not proportionally greater than PV-ICG, but may be variable depending on the size of the highly perfused interstitial volume, which mostly consists of brain, lungs, heart, liver, and kidneys.

When PV-ICG is overestimated, the relationship between these two volumes may be different. Thus, we should be concerned about the possible apparent overestimation of PV-ICG, because, as shown in this chapter, a considerable number of critically ill patients have the potential of PV-ICG overestimation, which leads to misinterpretation of the intravascular volume status.

8. IDVG and Overestimation of ICG-Derived Plasma Volume

We have been using indocyanine green (ICG) as an indicator of dilution volumetry for plasma volume (PV) measurement in either the intensive care unit (ICU) or the animal laboratory. Among the measurements, we had two patients who temporally had unusual large ICG-derived plasma volume (PV-ICG or Vd-ICG), even though none of the other clinical variables supported such a hypervolemic state (Ishihara et al. 1997).

Case Reports

Case 1

A very thin 68-year-old man was transferred to the general ICU 2h after he had suffered severe burn injury. Two years before he had lost his right lower extremity in a traffic accident. Second- and third-degree burns were present over nearly half of his total body surface area (TBSA). He received 1l lactated Ringer's solution before admission to the ICU. On arrival his arterial blood pressure was 50/28mmHg, hematocrit 50.1%, total plasma protein concentration 5.4g/100ml, and body weight 36.3kg. Fluid resuscitation with lactated Ringer's solution without colloidal solution was immediately started. During the first 6-h period, the patient received 3l lactated Ringer's solution. PV-ICG at 6h after admission was 2.63l (73ml/kg) (Table 8-1). However, clinical variables including IDVG did not support the presence of such hypervolemia but rather obviously that of hypovolemia. During the subsequent 12h, the patient further received 8.7l lactated Ringer's solution associated with 660ml fresh-frozen plasma. Judged from clinical variables such as arterial blood pressure, central venous pressure (CVP), urine output, hematocrit, and cardiac size on chest radiograph (cardiothoracic ratio, 50%–52%) as well as body weight change, intravascular volume in the subsequent 2 days became restored, associated with normal values of PV-ICG and IDVG. Both

TABLE 8-1. Pharmacokinetic and clinical variables in patient 1

	Postburn day			
	0	1	2	6
Body weight, kg	36.3	41.9	51.1	47.8
PV_{ICG}, l	2.67	1.78	1.90	2.60
PV_{ICG}, ml/kg[a]	73	49	52	71
Ke_{ICG}, /min	0.081	0.158	0.12	0.093
CL, ml/kg min	5	7	6	6
ICG, mg/100 ml[b]	1.02	1.20	1.15	0.98
AIC	−37	−28	−45	−52
IDVG, l	3.62	5.35	5.37	7.41
Pao_2 (kPa)/Fio_2	28.4/0.4	16.2/0.4	13.6/0.4	8.8/0.4
MAP, Torr	70	68	75	68
CVP, Torr	3	7	12	9
Urine flow, ml/h	91	224	245	114
Hematocrit, %	48.7	36.4	31.7	24.9
Protein, g/100 ml	3.6	3.6	3.3	5.4

PV_{ICG}, plasma volume determined by the ICG dilution method; ICG, indocyanine green; Ke_{ICG}, ICG disappearance rate; CL (clearance) = $PV_{ICG} \times Ke_{ICG}$; AIC, Akaike's Information Criterion for the PV_{ICG} determination; IDVG, initial distribution volume of glucose; FiO_2, fraction of inspired oxygen; MAP, mean arterial pressure; CVP, central venous pressure; protein, total plasma protein concentration

[a] Divided by body weight on admission to the ICU of 36.3 kg

[b] Plasma ICG concentration at 1 min postinfusion

Source: from Ishihara et al. (1997), p 11, table 1, with permission from Karger

PV-ICG and clinical variables including IDVG supported the presence of apparent hypervolemia on the sixth postburn day.

Case 2

A 47-year-old woman was transferred to the general ICU for reasons of acute respiratory distress on the second postoperative day following skin graft to her large burn skin area of the chest and abdomen. She had been staying in the ICU for stabilization before she underwent this operative procedure. The trachea was intubated immediately after this emergent admission. Her arterial blood pressure was 166/50 mmHg and CVP 12 mmHg. Arterial blood gases on a fraction of inspired oxygen (Fio_2) 1.0 were as follows: pH 7.36, $Paco_2$ 47 mmHg, Pao_2 38 mmHg. A clinical diagnosis of pulmonary edema was made from the observation that massive, foamy, yellow-orange airway secretions came out continuously from the tracheal tube and that she suffered from cardiovascular instability. Mechanical ventilatory support with positive end-expiratory pressure (PEEP) of 5 cmH_2O and a dopamine infusion of 3 μg/kg min were instituted. Pao_2 improved to 63 mmHg on a Fio_2 0.5 12 h later.

In the meantime, however, the patient became hypotensive: an arterial blood pressure of 70–80/36–40 mmHg was measured, associated with CVP 1 mmHg, which remained unchanged during the subsequent 2 days, even though a total of 1750 ml colloids with an increased dopamine infusion up to 10 μg/kg min were administered. A chest radiograph demonstrated a patchy, peripheral, nongravitational distribution of pulmonary edema without obvious cardiomegaly. Septal lines and pleural effusions were not seen. PV-ICG on the 3rd ICU day, namely, the 28th postburn day, was 4.63 l (77 ml/kg) without a simultaneous increase in IDVG (Table 8-2). ICG disappearance rate from plasma (KeICG) and ICG clearance were lower at that time compared to three other occasions in this patient. The plasma ICG concentration at 1 min after ICG administration on the 28th postburn day was found to decrease to 0.59 mg/100 ml as compared to 0.66 mg/100 ml on the 16th postburn day during her first ICU stay. Ventilatory support was required for 2 additional days because of slow recovery from respiratory distress, associated with considerable amounts of nonpurulent upper airway secretions. By the 5th ICU day, the pulmonary edema had clinically resolved. No additional colloids or blood products were administered. PV-ICG decreased to 3.52 l (58 ml/kg) on the 6th ICU day, namely the 31st postburn

TABLE 8-2. Pharmacokinetic and clinical variables in patient 2

	Before edema[c]	Before edema[c]	During edema	After edema
Postburn day	8	16	28	31
Body weight, kg	74.9	66.9	67.8	59.9
PV_{ICG}, l	2.81	3.38	4.63	3.52
PV_{ICG}, ml/kg[a]	47	56	77	58
Ke_{ICG}, /min	0.28	0.24	0.06	0.16
CL, ml/kg min	13	13	4	9
ICG, mg/100 ml[b]	0.62	0.66	0.59	0.75
AIC	−35	−40	−37	−39
IDVG, l	10.67	10.23	8.57	7.59
Pao_2 (kPa)/Fio_2	23/0.5	24/0.4	10/0.4	20/0.4
MAP, Torr	82	87	60	81
CVP, Torr	11	8	1	10
Urine flow, ml/h	115	120	89[d]	108
Hematocrit, %	27.3	26.6	22.0	28.7
Protein, g/100 ml	5.6	6.2	5.0	6.0

[a] Divided by preburn body weight of 60.0 kg
[b] Plasma ICG concentration at 1 min postinfusion
[c] During the previous admission to the ICU
[d] Associated with an infusion of furosemide of 4 mg/h
Source: from Ishihara et al. (1997), p 11, table 2, with permission from Karger

day, even though IDVG and body weight were further decreased. She was discharged from ICU on that day.

After we encountered these two patients, we decided to evaluate the relationship between IDVG and PV-ICG in different experimental and clinical pathological conditions. Valeri et al. (1973) reported overestimation of plasma volume derived by ^{125}I-serum albumin in 1973. According to their report, overestimation may occur in patients with traumatic injuries, carcinoma, cardiopulmonary disorders, and miscellaneous diagnoses. Presumably, vascular leak syndrome would have a major impact on the overestimation. The syndrome is characterized by an increase in vascular permeability and extravasation of fluids and proteins resulting in hypovolemia, hypoproteinemia, interstitial edema, and multiple organ failure (Baluna and Vitetta 1997). It can occur during various pathological conditions, such as sepsis, burns, trauma, surgery, and immunotherapy for cancer patients (Baluna and Vitetta 1997).

ICG is thought to stay in the intravascular compartment and to provide an estimate of plasma volume, because this dye binds to plasma proteins including albumin and α_1 lipoproteins (Henschen et al. 1993). In contrast, glucose cannot stay in the vascular compartment but distributes rapidly throughout the intra- and extravascular compartments when administered intravenously. Assuming that IDVG consistently reflects the central extracellular fluid (ECF) volume state, which is plasma volume plus the interstial fluid volume of higly perfused tissues, and that pharmacokinetic behavior of glucose in the capillary beds remains unchanged despite the presence of generalized capillary protein leakage, the PV-ICG/IDVG would help predict overestimation of plasma volume or the presence of leakage without chronologically repeated measurements, even though IDVG is not proportionally larger than plasma volume. We tested this hypothesis in experimental and clinical studies.

Experimental Endotoxin Injection

Sixteen mongrel dogs weighing 7.5–10.0 kg were divided randomly into two equal groups, one of which received lipopolysaccharide (LPS) to induce capillary leakage (Sakai et al. 1998). Both glucose (100 mg/kg) and ICG (0.5 mg/kg) were infused simultaneously through the left femoral venous catheter over 30 s. A 3.5-ml blood sample was drawn for determinations immediately before and 1, 2, 3, 4, 5, 7, 9, 11, 13, 15, and 20 min after administration. A total of approximately 50 ml was drawn during 20 min.

Following measurements and sampling for the pretreatment values, the dogs of the LPS group received LPS 0.3 mg/kg and those of the control group received isotonic saline IV. Four hours later, the second administration of indicators and blood sampling were performed in the same manner as described previously, as high vascular permeability has been reported to begin 4h after a small dose of injected endotoxin (Brigham et al. 1979). These data served as the posttreatment values. IDVG and PV-ICG were calculated as described in previous chapters.

A reduction in cardiac output (CO) following endotoxin injection was similar to that following saline injection in this study. However, endotoxin injection, even in a small dose, caused significant effects on the cardiovascular system, namely a decrease in mean arterial pressure, heart rate, and urine output as well as metabolic acidosis without an obvious reduction in CO as reported previously (D'Orio et al. 1989). Posttreatment Vd-ICG and IDVG decreased in the control group ($P < 0.05$). In contrast, the posttreatment IDVG in the LPS group decreased similarly to that observed in the control group ($P < 0.05$), but the corresponding Vd-ICG remained unchanged despite a considerable amount of blood sampling. As judged by very low plasma ICG concentrations immediately before the second ICG administration in this study, modification by the residual ICG in plasma of the pharmacokinetic behavior of ICG is negligible. Thus, overestimation of PV seems likely after endotoxin injection. These findings are comparable with a previous PV-ICG study using septic rats (Wang et al. 1993).

The Vd-ICG/IDVG ratio of the control group was 0.42 (range, 0.37–0.49), which remained unchanged following saline injection. The pretreatment ratio of the LPS group was 0.45 (0.45–0.51), which increased to 0.55 (0.47–0.74) following LPS injection ($P < 0.05$). The posttreatment ratio of the two groups was significantly different ($P < 0.01$) (Fig. 8-1). We conclude that the Vd-ICG/IDVG ratio can help identify capillary protein leakage induced by LPS injection.

Experimental Histamine Administration

Histamine is well known as a substance that characteristically increases the capillary permeability, probably via H_1-receptors (Putensen et al. 1992), by causing the endothelial cells to contact and separate at their boundaries, thus exposing the basement membrane, which is freely permeable to plasma proteins and water. Twenty-four mongrel dogs weighing 6.0–11.0kg were used for the experiments (Suzuki et al. 1999). Both glucose 100mg/kg and ICG 0.5mg/kg were infused simultaneously through the central venous line over 30s. Arterial blood samples were drawn for determining plasma glucose and ICG concentrations immediately before and at 1, 2, 3, 4, 5, 7, 9, 11, 15, 20, and 30min after the glucose and ICG infusions. These data served as the pretreatment values. Subsequently, histamine infusion was started at a rate of

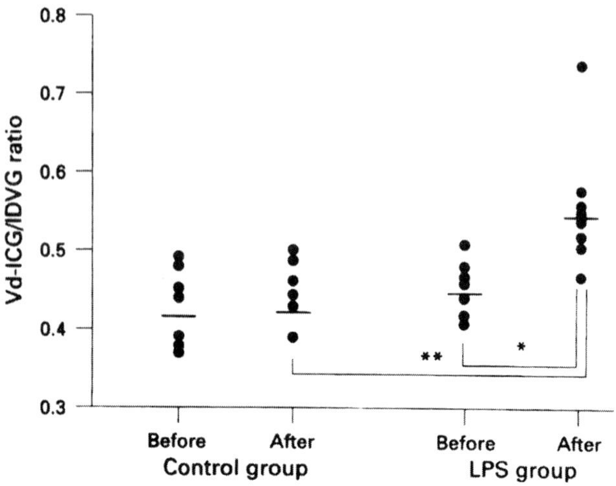

FIG. 8-1. Changes in the Vd-ICG/IDVG ratio in the control group and the LPS group. *Circles* indicate data of each dog with median (*horizontal bar*). *Vd-ICG*, plasma volume determined by the indocyanine green dilution method; *IDVG*, initial distribution volume of glucose; *LPS*, lipopolysaccharide; *Before*, before administration of isotonic saline or LPS; *After*, 4h after administration of isotonic saline or LPS; $^*P < 0.05$ compared with the pre-Vd-ICG ratio; $^{**}P < 0.01$ between the control and the LPS groups. (From Sakai et al. (1998), p 196, fig. 1, with permission from Oxford University Press)

50µg/kgh (histamine 50 group), or 100µg/kgh (histamine 100 group) in 8 dogs each. The remaining 8 dogs received normal saline solution instead of histamine. Ninety minutes after commencing the histamine or saline infusion, the second series of measurements and blood samplings was conducted as previously. These data served as the posttreatment values.

Assuming that the pretreatment Vd-ICG appropriately estimated PV, and that red blood cell volume remained unchanged during the experimental procedure despite blood sampling and potential mobilization of the red blood cells to the circulating blood from the spleen, the posttreatment PV (PV-post) (ml/kg) was also calculated from the changes in hematocrit (Hct) (%) and the pretreatment Vd-ICG (Vd-ICG-pre) (ml/kg) as follows:

$$\text{PV-post} = \text{RBC-pre} \times [100\text{-Hct-post}]/\text{Hct-post}]$$

$$\text{RBC-pre} = \text{Vd-ICG-pre} \times [\text{Hct-pre}/(100\text{-Hct-pre})]$$

where RBC-pre is the pretreatment volume of red blood cells (ml/kg), Hct-pre is pretreatment Hct, and Hct-post is posttreatment Hct.

Both hemoglobin (Hb) and Hct in the control group remained unchanged during the procedure, but posttreatment Hb and Hct of both histamine groups were significantly higher compared with the corresponding pretreatment values ($P < 0.05$). The posttreatment total plasma protein and albumin concentrations of both histamine groups decreased as compared with the corresponding pretreatment values ($P < 0.05$), but no differences were found among groups. Accordingly, an apparent capillary protein leakage would consistently occur in histamine groups.

No statistically significant reduction of Vd-ICG was observed following treatment in either of the histamine groups, even though the posttreatment Vd-ICG of the control group had decreased ($P < 0.05$) compared with the corresponding pretreatment value (Table 8-3).

The posttreatment PV calculated from the pretreatment Vd-ICG and changes of Hct were 45.7 ± 7.6 ml/kg, 38.7 ± 7.7 ml/kg, and 30.6 ± 8.2 ml/kg in the control, histamine 50, and histamine 100 groups, respectively. These posttreatment PV calculated were less than the posttreatment Vd-ICG in the two histamine groups ($P < 0.05$). Thus, the posttreatment Vd-ICG of histamine groups did not reflect the actual PV status. If further loss of red blood cells during the experimental procedure is ignored, then the posttreatment Vd-ICG overestimates PV by approximately 120% and 140% in the histamine 50 and histamine 100 groups, respectively.

Another important cardiovascular effect of histamine via both H_1- and H_2-receptors is capillary vasodilatation, which results in the trapping of a large amount of blood in the peripheral venules (Putensen et al. 1992). A further reduction of the central ECF volume is therefore possible due to trapping in addition to PV loss from the capillary beds.

The posttreatment Vd-ICG/IDVG ratio of the histamine 100 group increased compared with the corresponding pretreatment ratio ($P < 0.05$). A similar pattern was also observed in the histamine 50 group, even though the difference was not statistically significant (Fig. 8-2). The results suggest

TABLE 8-3. Changes in the indocyanine green and glucose dilutions (mean ± SD)

	Control group		Histamine 50 group		Histamine 100 group	
	Pre	Post	Pre	Post	Pre	Post
Vd-ICG (ml/kg)	45.9 ± 7.0	43.2 ± 5.8*	46.4 ± 7.1	44.8 ± 6.2	43.3 ± 6.3	40.6 ± 5.4
IDVG (ml/kg)	120.6 ± 19.4	118.4 ± 14.2	124.0 ± 24.4	115.4 ± 23.6*	117.0 ± 20.6	97.9 ± 17.5*
Vd-ICG/IDVG	0.38 ± 0.02	0.37 ± 0.06	0.38 ± 0.06	0.40 ± 0.06	0.37 ± 0.04	0.43 ± 0.06*

Pre, pretreatment values; Post, posttreatment values; Vd-ICG, distribution volume of indocyanine green; IDVG, initial distribution volume of glucose

* $P < 0.05$ compared with the pretreatment values

Source: from Suzuki et al. (1999), p 307, table 3, with permission from Springer

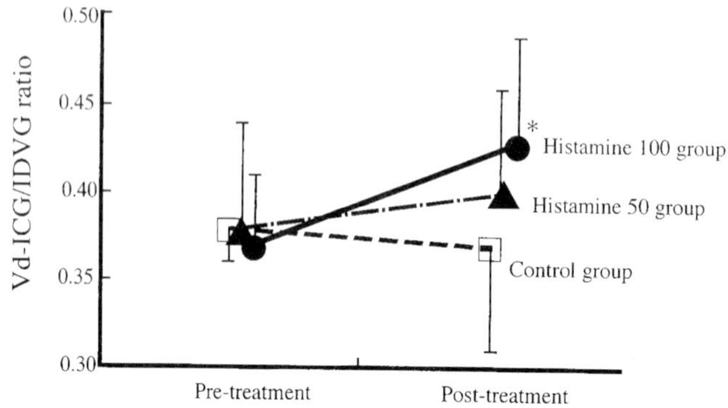

Fig. 8-2. Changes in the Vd-ICG/IDVG ratio (mean ± SD). *Vd-ICG*, distribution volume of indocyanine green; *IDVG*, initial distribution volume of glucose; $P < 0.05$ compared with the pretreatment value. (From Suzuki et al. (1999), p 307, fig. 1, with permission from Springer)

that Vd-ICG/IDVG ratio and IDVG are useful in evaluating the magnitude of the histamine-induced capillary protein leakage and hypovolemia.

Clinical Study of Burned Patients

Ten severely burned adult patients with or without inhalational injury admitted to the general ICU were enrolled (Ishihara et al. 1998a). Burn size ranged from 30% to 70% of the TBSA. All patients were admitted to the ICU within 24h postburn and required ventilatory support. A total of 30 comparisons were performed daily through the second postburn day. As part of their therapy, three patients required an infusion of vasoactive drugs including adrenaline and dopamine. Six patients had a flow-directed pulmonary artery catheter, and thermodilution CO was measured on six occasions immediately before each basal blood sampling for the determination of the two volumes within 24h postburn.

During the first 24-h postburn period, lactated Ringer's solution based on the Parkland formula was administered to achieve urine output more than 1ml/kg/h. Subsequently, a glucose solution (4.3%–14%) for routine nutritional support with or without enteral nutrition was added to the infusion of lactated Ringer's solution and fresh-frozen plasma. None of the patients received a continuous insulin infusion. Both 25ml glucose, 20% (5g) and 10ml ICG (25mg) were infused simultaneously over 30s through the central venous catheter. Serial blood samples were obtained through an indwelling femoral catheter immediately before and 1, 2, 3, 5, 7, 9, and 11min after the completion of both ICG and glucose infusions. Measurements were made three times: during fluid resuscitation within 24h postburn, at 24h postburn, and at 48h postburn. Calculated values were presented based on the basis of the reported preburn body weight.

The median IDVG and PV-ICG within 24h postburn were 78 (range, 58–113) ml/kg and 29 (22–74) ml/kg, respectively. The former increased at 24h postburn ($P < 0.05$), but the latter remained unchanged throughout the study period. Although no correlation was found between these two volumes within 24h postburn ($r = 0.46$), a linear correlation was found between these two volumes at 24h postburn ($r = 0.88$, $n = 10$, $P < 0.001$) and at 48h postburn ($r = 0.93$, $n = 10$, $P < 0.001$). The Ke-ICG was increased at 24 and 48h postburn compared to the time within 24h postburn ($P < 0.05$). The disappearance rate of glucose from plasma (Ke-glucose) remained unchanged throughout the study period.

Body weight increased at 24 and 48h postburn compared to that within 24h postburn ($P < 0.01$, respectively) (Table 8-4). Although hematocrit decreased at 24 and 48h postburn compared to that within 24h postburn, a statistically significant reduction was observed only at 48h postburn ($P < 0.01$). Other clinical variables, including mean arterial pressure (MAP), CVP, and total plasma protein concentration, remained unchanged during the study period. CO within 24h postburn correlated with IDVG ($r = 0.83$, $n = 6$,

TABLE 8-4. Fluid volumes and pharmacokinetic variables during the early postburn period

	Within 24h	24h	48h
Weight (kg)	73.2 (36.3–82.9)	80.1 (41.9–98.3)*	82.4 (51.1–96.6)**
Hematocrit (%)	47.8 (40.6–57.9)	44.4 (27.5–53.8)	38.3 (24.5–51.8)**
Plasma protein (g/100ml)	3.6 (2.4–4.6)	3.6 (3.0–4.2)	3.9 (3.3–4.6)
Plasma glucose (mmol/l)	8.6 (5.8–13.5)	8.4 (6.1–11.8)	8.9 (5.5–10.8)
IDVG (ml/kg)[a]	78 (58–113)	90 (76–147)	95 (73–148)
Ke-glucose (/min)	0.08 (0.04–0.11)	0.09 (0.07–0.11)	0.09 (0.07–0.11)
PV-ICG (ml/kg)[a]	29 (22–74)	29 (26–49)	33 (27–52)
Ke-ICG (/min)	0.23 (0.08–0.31)	0.32 (0.16–0.60)*	0.34 (0.12–0.65)*
PV-ICG/IDVG ratio	0.36 (0.25–0.74)	0.33 (0.27–0.38)**	0.35 (0.30–0.42)

Plasma protein, total plasma protein concentration; plasma glucose, plasma glucose present before glucose challenge; IDVG, initial distribution volume of glucose; Ke-glucose, disappearance rate of glucose from plasma; PV-ICG, ICG derived plasma volume; Ke-ICG, disappearance rate of ICG from plasma

[a] Based on reported preburn body weight

* $P < 0.05$ versus within 24h; ** $P < 0.01$ versus within 24h

Source: modified from Ishihara et al. (1998a), p 528, table 3, and p 529, table 4, with permission from Elsevier

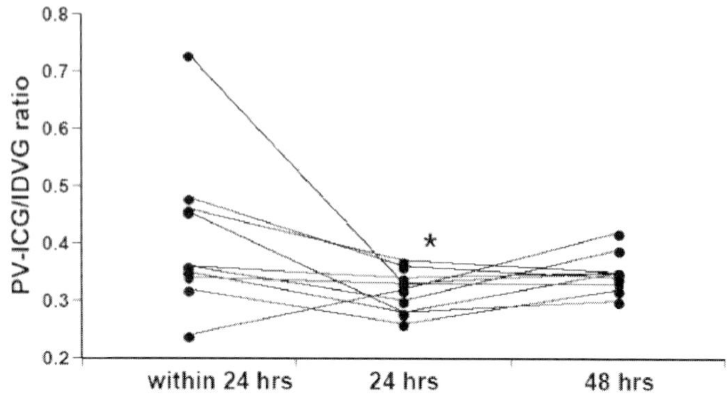

FIG. 8-3. Changes in the PV-ICG/IDVG ratio in the early postburn period. *PV-ICG*, plasma volume determined by the indocyanine green (ICG) dilution method; *IDVG*, initial distribution volume of glucose; *$P < 0.01$ versus within 24h. (Modified from Ishihara et al. (1998a), p 528, fig. 1, with permission from Elsevier)

$P < 0.05$). However, no correlation was observed between PV-ICG and CO ($r = 0.20$). Although the median PV-ICG/IDVG ratio was 0.36 (0.25–0.74) within 24h postburn day, four patients had a ratio greater than 0.45 within 24h postburn, which was not observed in subsequent measurements (Fig. 8-3).

Plasma protein concentration reaches its minimum at 8–10h postburn, leading to maximum edema formation in the nonburned tissues at this time (Dembling 1987). By 24 hours postburn, the increased vascular permeability to protein has largely returned to normal (Pruitt 1978). Thus, these pathophysiological processes would support our findings, even though two of ten patients were evaluated within 6h postburn and the PV-ICG/IDVG ratio within 24h postburn was not consistently high compared to the ratio at 24h postburn. The results suggest that simultaneous measurement of PV-ICG and IDVG would help identify the generalized capillary protein leakage early after burns.

Clinical Study of Septic Patients

A total of 12 septic patients and 16 patients with acute myocardial infarction (AMI) were enrolled (Ishihara et al. 2000c). Sepsis was diagnosed from the criteria proposed by a consensus conference sponsored by the American College of Chest Physicians and the Society of Critical Care Medicine (Bone et al. 1992). AMI patients served as controls, and none of them had any apparent underlying pathology causing protein capillary leakage. Study of the septic patients was performed on day 1 when the patients met the criteria of sepsis in the ICU, whereas the study of the AMI patients was performed on the day of admission to the ICU immediately after percutaneous coronary intervention. Some patients of either group received an infusion of vasoactive drugs such as dobutamine or an infusion of insulin. In addition, three AMI patients required cardiac support with an intraaortic balloon pump. Two septic patients required continuous hemodiafiltration. Both glucose and ICG were administered and measured in the same manner as described in the burn study. Thermodilution CO was measured in two septic patients and all AMI patients.

Fluid volumes studied in both groups are presented in Table 8-5. Pharmacokinetic and routine clinical variables for each septic patient are presented in Table 8-6. Linear correlations were determined between PV-ICG and IDVG in the two patient groups, that is, for the septic patients ($r^2 = 0.47$, $P < 0.025$) and for the AMI patients ($r^2 = 0.78$, P .014 0.01), respectively (Fig. 8-4). Although IDVG of the two patient groups was not statistically different, PV-ICG in the septic patients was greater than that in the AMI patients ($P < 0.01$). Consequently, the PV-ICG/IDVG ratio in the septic patients was higher than that in the AMI patients ($P < 0.01$). Eight of the 12 septic patients had a ratio of more than 0.45, which was not observed in any of the AMI patients (Fig. 8-5). Five of the 12 septic patients died of complications from sepsis less than 4 days after the study was performed. The remaining patients recovered from sepsis and were discharged from the ICU. The PV-ICG/IDVG ratio of the 7 survivors on the day of discharge from the ICU was significantly lower than

TABLE 8-5. Comparison of pharmacokinetic variables between the two patient groups

	Sepsis (n = 12)	AMI (n = 16)	*P*
Plasma glucose (mmol/l)	7.8 (3.2–13.9)	8.1 (5.1–18.0)	NS
AIC for glucose curve	−20.4 (−31.7–16.3)	−24.7 (−41.9–18.1)	NS
IDVG (ml/kg)	112 (85–182)	118 (76–153)	NS
Ke-gl (/min)	0.09 (0.04–0.12)	0.06 (0.03–0.08)	<0.01
AIC for ICG curve	−44.5 (−61.4–29.3)	−42.2 (−64.0–27.7)	NS
PV-ICG (ml/kg)	53 (39–107)	42.7 (27–56)	<0.01
Ke-ICG (/min)	0.11 (0.01–0.36)	0.16 (0.09–0.25)	NS
PV-ICG/IDVG ratio	0.47 (0.29–0.63)	0.38 (0.30–0.43)	<0.01

Data are presented as median (range) values

AMI, acute myocardial infarction; plasma glucose, plasma glucose presented immediately before glucose challenge; AIC, Akaike's information criterion; IDVG, initial distribution volume of glucose; Ke-gl, glucose disappearance rate from plasma; PV-ICG, plasma volume determined by the indocyanine green (ICG) dilution method; Ke-ICG, ICG disappearance rate from plasma; NS, not significant

Source: from Ishihara (2000c), p. 623, table 4, with permission from Lippincott Williams & Wilkins

TABLE 8-6. Pharmacokinetic and routine clinical variables in each septic patient

Patient no.	PV-ICG (ml/kg)	Ke-ICG (/min)	IDVG (ml/kg)	Ke-gl (/min)	Ratio	Incremental BW (kg)	MAP (mm Hg)	CVP (mm Hg)	Hct (%)	Protein (g/100 ml)
1	39	0.01	104	0.07	0.38	1.9	106	8	24.6	5.6
2	60	0.10	127	0.10	0.47	6.3	45	7	24.8	5.5
3	46	0.26	101	0.07	0.46	1.2	56	4	37.6	5.5
4	68	0.36	147	0.05	0.46	1.2	79	11	21.4	4.8
5	57	0.10	118	0.11	0.48	8.8	76	6	25.9	4.9
6	39	0.15	85	0.09	0.46	−1.5	74	14	25.1	5.2
7	52	0.07	182	0.04	0.29	0.5	96	11	25.8	6.4
8	70	0.21	134	0.09	0.52	0.2	84	9	21.5	4.8
9	107	0.13	170	0.12	0.63	5.7	40	10	26.7	3.6
10	54	0.06	108	0.10	0.52	9.2	83	10	24.1	4.6
11	51	0.08	105	0.08	0.49	3.4	80	9	29.4	6.5
12	43	0.16	98	0.11	0.44	2.8	94	9	33.5	4.2

PV-ICG, plasma volume determined by the indocyanine green (ICG) dilution method; Ke-ICG, ICG disappearance rate from plasma; IDVG, initial distribution volume of glucose; Ke-gl, glucose disappearance rate from plasma; Ratio, PV-ICG/IDVG ratio; Incremental BW, increased body weight above the reported basal body weight before admission to the intensive care unit; MAP, mean arterial pressure; CVP, central venous pressure; Hct, hematocrit; Protein, total plasma protein concentration

Source: from Ishihara et al. (2000c), p 622, table 3, with permission from Lippincott Williams & Wilkins

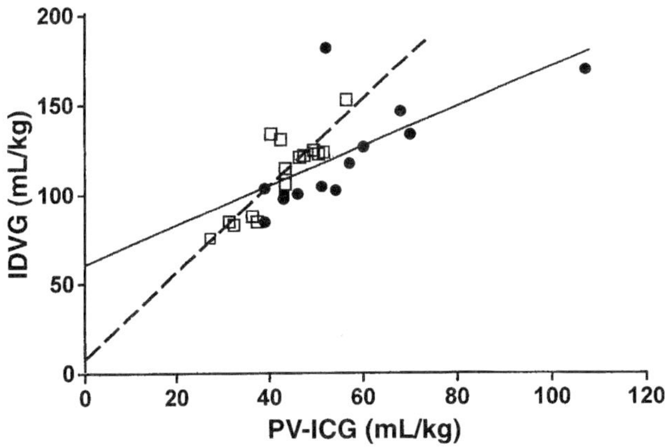

FIG. 8-4. Relationship between PV-ICG and IDVG in septic patients and acute myocardial infarction patients. *Circles*, each point for septic patients; *solid line*, regression line for the septic patients, i.e., $Y = 1.1X + 59$; $r^2 = 0.47$; $n = 12$; $P < 0.01$. *Squares*, each point for acute myocardial infarction patients; *dashed line*, regression line for the acute myocardial infarction patients, i.e., $y = 2.4x + 3.5$; $r^2 = 0.78$; $n = 16$; $P < 0.01$. *PV-ICG*, plasma volume determined by the indocyanine green dilution method; *IDVG*, initial distribution volume of glucose. (From Ishihara et al. (2000c), p 623, fig. 1, with permission from Lippincott Williams & Wilkins)

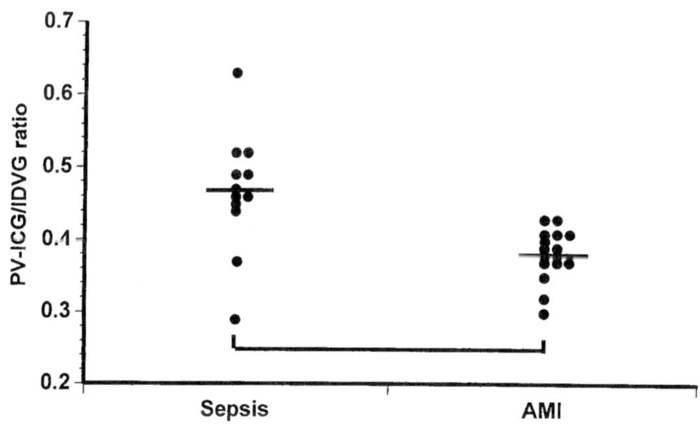

FIG. 8-5. PV-ICG/IDVG ratio in septic patients and acute myocardial infarction (AMI) patients. *Circles*, data for each patient with median (*horizontal bar*). $P < 0.01$ between the two patient groups. *PV-ICG*, plasma volume determined by the indocyanine green dilution method; *IDVG*, initial distribution volume of glucose. (From Ishihara et al. (2000c), p 624, fig. 2, with permission from Lippincott Williams & Wilkins)

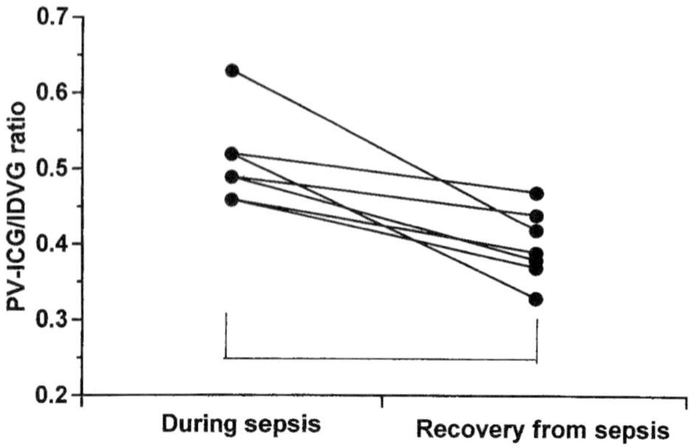

FIG. 8-6. Changes in PV-ICG/IDVG ratio in seven survivors of sepsis. $P = 0.01$ between two different times. *PV-ICG*, plasma volume determined by the indocyanine green dilution method; *IDVG*, initial distribution volume of glucose; *During sepsis*, on day 1, when patients met the criteria for sepsis; *Recovery from sepsis*, on the day of discharge from the ICU. (From Ishihara et al. (2000c), p 624, fig. 3, with permission from Lippincott Williams & Wilkins)

that on day 1 of sepsis ($P < 0.01$) (Fig. 8-6). The PV-ICG/IDVG ratio in the septic patients correlated inversely with total plasma protein concentration ($r^2 = 0.46$, $P < 0.025$) and mean arterial pressure ($r^2 = 0.42$, $P < 0.025$). No such correlations were determined in the AMI patients. The ratio of survivors from sepsis on the day of discharge from the ICU was decreased and became similar to the ratio observed in the AMI patients.

Although IDVG in the septic and AMI patient groups was not different, the disappearance rate of glucose from plasma in the septic patients was significantly higher than in AMI patients. Consequently, plasma glucose clearance rate in the septic patients was apparently augmented, as reported previously (Wolfe et al. 1977; Chinkes et al. 1995), suggesting that glucose in the central compartment moves rapidly into the peripheral compartment by insulin-like activity or by an unknown mechanism independent of distribution volume. Chinkes et al. (1995) clearly demonstrated that the increased plasma glucose clearance rate in sepsis is caused by an increased exchange between the plasma and interstitial fluid and is not related to glucose transport into the cells. Our results indicate that simultaneous measurement of these two volumes can help identify generalized capillary protein leakage as well as fluid volume status without chronologically repeated measurements in septic patients.

Clinical Study of Cardiac Surgical Patients

Twenty-four consecutive postcardiac surgical patients postoperatively admitted to the general ICU were enrolled (Ishihara et al. 2002). Surgical procedures consisted of coronary artery bypass grafting (15), aortic or mitral valve surgery (7), and total aortic arch replacements using cardiopulmonary bypass (2). Fluid volumes were assessed postoperatively twice: immediately after admission to the ICU and between 9 and 11 A.M. on the first postoperative day. ICG (25 mg) in 10 ml glucose 50% (5 g) solution was administered as a single bolus injection through the proximal port of a flow-directed pulmonary artery catheter. Serial blood samples were obtained as performed in the same manner as described in the burn study.

A glucose-containing crystalloid solution, glucose 4.3%, was infused continuously for routine postoperative fluid management through a central venous line using an electric pump at a constant rate: 1.5 ml/kg h. Lactated Ringer's solution, plasma protein fraction, and/or packed red blood cells were further administered as clinically required. Additionally, as part of therapy, all but 1 occasion required infusions of dopamine, dobutamine, and/or norepinephrine. Five occasions required intraaortic balloon pumping, and 19 occasions required an infusion of insulin ranging from 0.5 to 5.0 unit/h. Although all patients required mechanical ventilatory support without applying positive endexpiratory pressure (PEEP) immediately after admission to the ICU, the trachea had been extubated before the second determination in 19 patients, and these patients were discharged from the ICU on the first postoperative day. One patient had obvious cardiovascular instability during data collection on the first postoperative day. Thus, comparison of PV-ICG and IDVG was done on the remaining 47 determinations. Thermodilution CO was not obtained in 1 patient on the first postoperative day due to failure of the CO monitor.

Fluid volume status on the 2 study days is shown in Table 8-7. Body weight and routine cardiovascular variables including CO remained statistically unchanged. PV-ICG and IDVG on the first postoperative day were higher than those on the operative day ($P < 0.001$ and $P = 0.001$, respectively). The Hct value on the first postoperative day was lower than that on the operative day ($P < 0.001$). IDVG correlated linearly with PV-ICG on the operative day ($r = 0.68$, $n = 24$, $P < 0.001$) and on the first postoperative day ($r = 0.78$, $n = 23$, $P < 0.001$) (Fig. 8-7). IDVG correlated linearly with PV-ICG using all data ($r = 0.74$. $n = 47$, $P < 0.001$). The mean PV-ICG/IDVG ratio was 0.38 ± 0.05, ranging from 0.27 to 0.48. Four recordings had a PV-ICG/ IDVG ratio higher than 0.45: 0.46, 0.46, 0.47, and 0.48, respectively.

TABLE 8-7. Daily fluid volume status

Variable	Operative day ($n = 24$)	First postoperative day ($n = 23$)	P value
BW (kg)	59.5 ± 10.6	58.8 ± 10.3	NS
Hct (%)	34.7 ± 5.8	29.8 ± 3.7	<0.001
PAWP (mm Hg)	8 ± 3	9 ± 5	NS
CVP (mm Hg)	5 ± 2	6 ± 3	NS
CO-TD (L/min)	4.8 ± 1.3	5.2 ± 1.1	NS
PV-ICG (L)	2.3 ± 0.5	2.6 ± 0.5	<0.001
PV-PDD (L)	2.3 ± 0.8	2.7 ± 0.7	0.007
IDVG (L)	6.2 ± 1.3	7.0 ± 1.3	0.001
PV-ICG/IDVG ratio	0.38 ± 0.06	0.38 ± 0.05	NS
PV-PDD/IDVG ratio	0.39 ± 0.12	0.39 ± 0.07	NS

Values are presented as mean ± SD

BW, body weight; Hct, hematocrit; PAWP, pulmonary artery wedge pressure; CVP, central venous pressure; CO-TD, continuous thermodilution cardiac output; PV-ICG, the conventional indocyanine green dilution-derived plasma volume requiring repeated blood sampling; PV-PDD, pulse dye densitometry-derived plasma volume; IDVG, initial distribution volume of glucose

Source: from Ishihara et al. (2002), p 784, table 2, with permission from Lippincott Williams & Wilkins

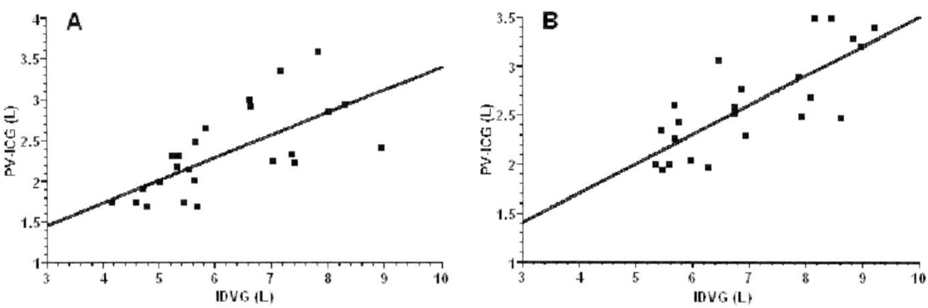

FIG. 8-7. Relationship between initial distribution volume of glucose (*IDVG*) and volume determined by the conventional indocyanine green dilution method (*PV-ICG*) in post-cardiac surgical patients postoperatively on the operative day (**A**) and on the first post-operative day (**B**). $Y = 0.28X + 0.6$; $r = 0.68$; $n = 24$; $P = 0.00023$ (**A**); $Y = 0.3X + 0.5$; $r = 0.78$; $n = 23$; $P = 0.000013$ (**B**). (From Ishihara et al. (2002), p 784, fig. 1, with permission from Lippincott Williams & Wilkins)

Cardiac surgery with cardiopulmonary bypass is generally believed to be associated with altered vascular endothelial integrity and albumin leakage from the intravascular compartment (Boldt 2000), suggesting that overestimation of PV-ICG can occur after cardiac surgery as well. However, our results suggest that most of the PV-ICG measurements are accurate, in contrast to our results early after esophagectomy in which approximately 30% of PV-ICG measurements were associated with a PV-ICG/IDVG higher than

0.45 (Ishihara et al. 2000c). Interestingly, our two postcardiac surgical patients who underwent prolonged surgical procedures that lasted more than 10 h associated with massive intraoperative hemorrhage did not have a ratio higher than 0.45. Assuming that preoperative body weight is 60 kg, associated with the normal IDVG of 120 ml/kg, and the threshold ratio of the leakage is set at 0.45, the PV-ICG/IDVG ratio of 0.48, which was the highest ratio in our postcardiac surgery study, would yield overestimation of PV-ICG by approximately 150 ml. Presumably the overestimation can be clinically negligible, even if present. Considering our findings, PV-ICG measurement by using the traditional blood sampling method is accurate early after cardiac surgery but not after esophagectomy.

Clinical Study Early After Induction of Propofol/ Fentanyl Anesthesia

Thirteen patients scheduled for general anesthesia were recruited to participate in this study (Mi et al. 2003). None of the patients had any history or signs of cardiopulmonary diseases (ASA physical status 1) or inflammatory diseases. PV-ICG and IDVG were assessed twice: at 15 min before induction of anesthesia (preinduction data) and at 15 min after the start of induction of anesthesia (postinduction data). ICG (25 mg) in 10 ml glucose 50% (5 g) solution was administered as a single bolus injection through the cubital vein route over 10 s. Fifteen minutes after the first measurement, anesthesia was induced with fentanyl and propofol IV. Vecuronium 0.1 mg/kg was given to facilitate tracheal intubation. Fifteen minutes after the start of induction, the second administration of ICG and glucose followed by arterial blood sampling, and measurements was performed in the same manner as described previously.

Estimated blood volume derived by ICG dilution (BV-ICG) was calculated from BV-ICG and Hct (%) as follows:

$$\text{BV-ICG} = \text{PV-ICG}/(1 - \text{Hct}/100)$$

Estimated red blood cell volume (RCV-ICG) was also calculated from BV-ICG and PV-ICG:

$$\text{RCV-ICG} = \text{PV-ICG} \times \text{Hct}/100/(1 - \text{Hct}/100)$$

Percentile increase in PV was calculated as follows (Brauer et al. 2002):

$$(\text{Hb}_0 - \text{Hb}_p)/\text{Hb}_p \div (1 - \text{Hct}_0/100) \times 100\%$$

where Hct_0 represents Hct at preinduction and Hb_0 and Hb_p represent the Hb at preinduction and at postinduction, respectively.

The mean PV-ICG, BV-ICG, and RCV-ICG after induction of anesthesia increased significantly by an average of 15.3%, 14.1%, and 10.6%, respectively ($P < 0.001$ for both PV-ICG and BV-ICG, $P = 0.007$ for RCV-ICG) (Table 8-8). PV-ICG at postinduction increased in ten patients and remained almost unchanged in three patients (Fig. 8-8). Percentile increase in PV based on changes in Hb and Hct was 4%. Consequently, an 11% possible overestimation in PV-ICG was obtained. IDVG remained unchanged. The PV-ICG/IDVG ratio before induction ranged from 0.31 to 0.48, with only one patient being greater than 0.45. After induction, seven recordings had a PV-ICG/IDVG ratio above 0.45 with two above 0.50. Hct values and concentration of Hb and total plasma protein at postinduction in each patient decreased by an average of 2.9%, 2.2%, and 2.3%, respectively, as compared with preinduction values ($P < 0.05$). The mean Ke-ICG before induction was 0.27 ± 0.03/min (range, 0.22–0.32), which indicates that almost all the administered ICG (99.8%) had been cleared from plasma immediately before the second injection of ICG, even in the patient with the lowest Ke-ICG (0.22).

TABLE 8-8. Measured and calculated variables before and after induction of anesthesia ($n = 13$)

	Preinduction	Postinduction	*P* value
PV-ICG (l)	2.29 ± 0.38 (1.82–2.90)	2.64 ± 0.31 (2.00–3.11)	<0.001
PV-ICG/BSA (l/m^2)	1.43 ± 0.20 (1.15–1.79)	1.67 ± 0.18 (1.27–1.97)	<0.001
RCV-ICG (l)	1.33 ± 0.25 (1.00–1.99)	1.47 ± 0.30 (1.03–2.14)	0.007
RCV-ICG/BSA (l/m^2)	0.83 ± 0.11 (0.62–1.04)	0.92 ± 0.16 (0.64–1.12)	0.008
BV-ICG (l)	3.61 ± 0.56 (3.04–4.90)	4.12 ± 0.53 (3.08–5.25)	<0.001
BV-ICG/BSA (l/m^2)	2.26 ± 0.26 (1.95–2.78)	2.59 ± 0.29 (1.95–3.04)	0.002
Ke-ICG (/min)	0.27 ± 0.03 (0.22–0.32)	0.21 ± 0.03 (0.16–0.25)	<0.001
IDVG (l)	5.75 ± 0.66 (4.69–6.70)	5.60 ± 0.86 (4.07–7.45)	0.548
IDVG/BSA (l/m^2)	3.61 ± 0.41 (3.02–4.19)	3.52 ± 0.44 (2.70–4.26)	0.495
Ke-glucose (/min)	0.09 ± 0.02 (0.07–0.14)	0.09 ± 0.02 (0.08–0.14)	0.359
PV-ICG/IDVG ratio	0.40 ± 0.05 (0.31–0.48)	0.48 ± 0.06 (0.41–0.65)	0.006
Hematocrit (%)	36.6 ± 3.7 (27.0–41.0)	35.6 ± 3.8 (26.5–40.7)	0.003
Hemoglobin (g/100 ml)	12.7 ± 1.7 (8.4–15.1)	12.4 ± 1.8 (8.1–14.6)	0.034
TP (g/100 ml)	6.6 ± 0.5 (6.0–7.5)	6.4 ± 0.5 (5.7–7.4)	<0.001

Data expressed as mean ± SD (range)
PV-ICG, plasma volume determined by indocyanine green; RCV-ICG, red cell volume calculated from PV-ICG and hematocrit; BV-ICG, estimated blood volume calculated from PV-ICG and hematocrit; Ke-ICG, ICG disappearance rate from plasma; IDVG, initial distribution volume of glucose; Ke-glucose, glucose disappearance rate from plasma; BSA, body surface area; TP, total plasma protein
Source: from Mi et al. Anesth Analg 2003;97:1421–1427 (p 1424, table 2), with permission from Lippincott Williams & Wilkins

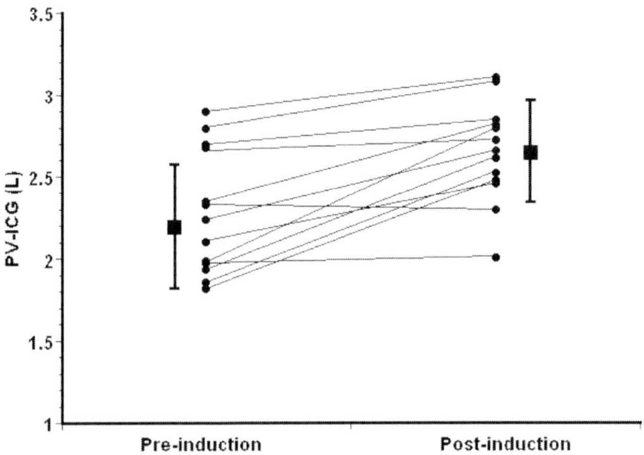

FIG. 8-8. Changes in plasma volume determined by the indocyanine green dilution method (*PV-ICG*) in each patient before and after induction of anesthesia. *Vertical lines* indicate mean and SD before and after induction of anesthesia. (From Mi et al. (2003), p 1424, fig. 1, with permission from Lippincott Williams & Wilkins)

Assuming that RCV-ICG is a reference of erythrocyte volume, it should remain unchanged regardless of changes in either arterial Hct or PV-ICG, provided there is no gain or loss of erythrocytes. As indicated by a formula for indirect calculation of RCV-ICG from PV-ICG and Hct, an apparent increase in PV-ICG associated with a small decrease in Hct yielded an erroneous increase in RCV-ICG after induction of anesthesia in our study. The result further supports the hypothesis that possible overestimation of PV-ICG occurs during the early period after anesthetic induction. Although the underlying mechanism of the overestimation in PV-ICG has not been fully clarified, either increased capillary exchange surface area, increased amount of unbound ICG, and/or increased capillary permeability may play a role. It remains unclear how long the overestimation in PV-ICG after induction will remain or how the extent will vary chronologically during anesthesia. Avram et al. (2000) observed no differences between PV-ICG values at 1.5–2 h after induction of anesthesia. In some clinical practices, we measured PV-ICG and arterial Hct, and thus RCV-ICG. We found that the RCV-ICG values at 1.5–2 h after anesthetic induction were significantly smaller than those estimated during a short period after anesthetic induction, although no obvious blood loss was observed between the two measurements. These phenomena imply that the overestimation during anesthesia changes over time. We conclude that possible overestimation of PV-ICG occurs during a definable period of time after propofol anesthetic induction.

Detection of Overestimation of ICG-Derived Plasma Volume

Protein leakage from capillary beds may affect intravascular pharmacokinetic behavior of ICG because this dye binds to plasma proteins (Henschen et al. 1993). Presumably, two different results would occur as a result of the leakage. First, the administered ICG would be distributed throughout a space larger than the actual intravascular space (Fig. 8-9, lower part). Second, elimination of ICG from plasma would be further augmented through tissues other than the liver (Fig. 8-9, upper part). The reported rate of loss of albumin to the extravascular space is approximately 5%/h even in healthy humans and it may be augmented by more than 300% in patients with septic shock (Fleck et al. 1985). Hahn (2005) stated that a sampling period less than 10 min is too short to evaluate capillary protein leakage. Additionally, Imai et al. (2000) reported that ICG-pulse dye densitometry (ICG-PDD), utilizing the dye concentrations between 2.5 and 5.5 min after the mean transit time of administered ICG, can provide the intravascular volume state independently of permeability of vascular beds to albumin. According to the results of our experimental and clinical studies, an apparent increase in Ke-ICG was not observed in the presence of underlying capillary leak pathology. In contrast, an erroneously large distribution volume of ICG was obtained from both the traditional blood sampling method, as described in this chapter, and ICG-PDD, as shown in Fig. 8-10. Therefore, overestimation of ICG-derived intra-

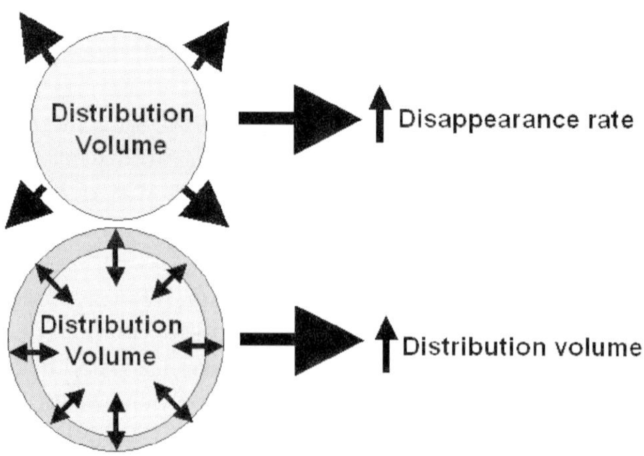

Fig. 8-9. Possible pharmacokinetic behavior during protein capillary leakage. *Upper part*: increased disappearance rate from plasma without an increase in distribution volume; *lower part*: increased distribution volume without an increase in disappearance rate from plasma

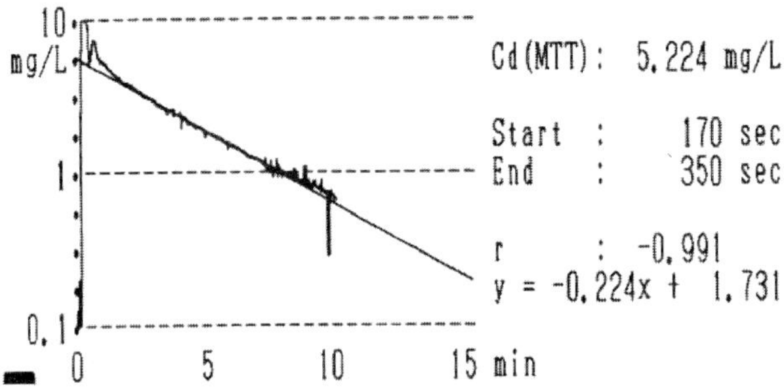

FIG. 8-10. Overestimation of circulating blood volume derived from either ICG pulse dye densitometry or the conventional blood sampling method. Note: an apparent overestimation of circulating blood volume was recorded in a 71-year-old man (height, 155 cm; body weight, 45 kg) requiring intraaortic balloon pumping for 30 h after onset of acute myocardial infarction before emergency coronary artery bypass grafting. Clinical variables and symptoms as well as IDVG [6.01 (133 ml/kg)] did not support obvious fluid accumulation in this patient. ICG 25 mg was injected through the right internal jugular vein. The regression line derived from ICG-pulse dye densitometry was back-extrapolated to the mean transit time (MTT) for the first circulation curve of ICG [*Cd (MTT)*] as described in Chapter 1. Circulating blood volume was calculated from dose (25 mg) divided by Cd (MTT) (5.224 mg/l). Volume was 4.79 l (106 ml/kg). Circulating blood volume was also calculated from PV-ICG using the conventional blood sampling method (3.57 l) and hematocrit (28.1%). Volume was 4.97 l (110 ml/kg); PV-ICG/IDVG ratio was 0.59

vascular volume would occur, even if sampling period were relatively short. Presumably, the magnitude of overestimation in PV-ICG would not directly reflect the rate of loss of albumin to the extravascular space.

Our clinical studies demonstrate that apparent overestimation of PV-ICG is detected in burned, septic, or postesophagectomy patients (Fig. 8-11). Possible overestimation was observed early after induction of propofol/fentanyl anesthesia. Apparent overestimation was not found early after cardiac surgery or early after percutaneous coronary intervention in AMI patients. Interestingly, AMI patients whose condition was severe enough to require mechanical cardiac support such as intraaortic balloon pumping had a ratio less than 0.45 immediately after percutaneous intervention. Additionally, the reported PV-ICG value of the AMI patients in the absence of percutaneous coronary intervention was similar to the value of healthy volunteers (44 ± 5 ml/kg), whether or not the patients survived (Da Luz et al. 1974). These findings allow speculation that the protein leakage in either surgical or medical cardiac patients during the first day of acute illness would not be severe enough to produce apparent overestimation of PV-ICG. However, when acute illness was not resolved within 24 h after its onset, overestimation may occur (see Fig. 8-10). According to the results of the histamine study (Suzuki et al. 1999), the magnitude of the overestimation would be correlated

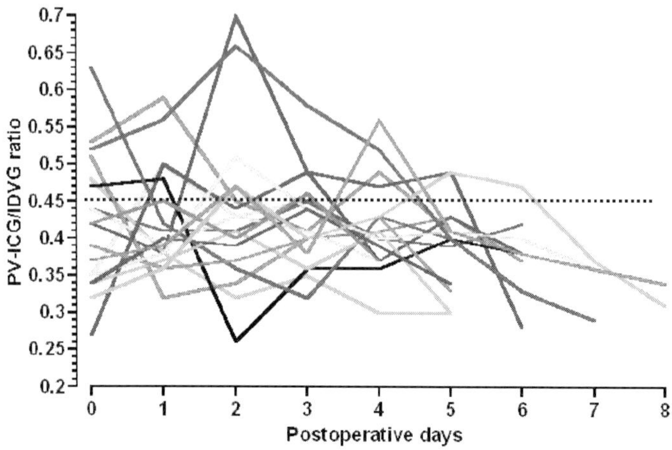

FIG. 8-11. Daily changes of the PV-ICG/IDVG in 19 surgical patients following esophagectomy Note: possible overestimation of PV-ICG may occur approximately through to the fifth postoperative day

with the PV-ICG/IDVG ratio. Thus, we believe our method can detect the overestimation induced by leakage. Comparative measurement using ^{35}Cr-labeled red cells may allow confirmation of our assumption.

Redistribution of blood from the central to the peripheral compartment may also occur in endotoxemia and peripheral pooling of blood (D'Orio et al. 1989; Imu and Charlson 1993), which would yield a high PV-ICG/IDVG ratio as well, regardless of the presence or absence of protein leakage. Contribution of redistribution is discussed in the next chapter.

The chronological changes in Hct, total plasma protein, albumin concentration, urine volume, and hemodynamic variables indirectly indicate capillary protein leakage and associated hypovolemia. However, it is difficult to evaluate these changes with a single measurement of these variables or under the influence of various pathologies as well as fluid therapy in critically ill patients. In addition, the hemodynamic variables do not change consistently until the development of obvious hypovolemia. Measurement of the ratio would provide more evidence-based fluid therapy. According to our experience, approximately 10% of the ICU patients including both surgical and nonsurgical patients had a PV-ICG/IDVG ratio higher than 0.45 (Ishihara et al. 1999). However, the combined measurement would require approximately 1h from the start of sampling to completion of calculation of both distribution volumes. Thus, further advanced technology is required for clinically applicable detection of the overestimation.

9. IDVG and Redistribution of Fluid

In previous chapters, we have demonstrated that the initial distribution volume of glucose (IDVG) represents the central extracellular fluid (ECF) volume. However, it is not clear whether IDVG consistently reflects the state of the central ECF volume even when redistribution of fluid occurs in the absence of fluid gain or loss. As indicated by a report in which application of positive end-expiratory pressure induced a considerable decrease in cardiac output (CO) without affecting indocyanine green (ICG)-derived plasma volume (PV-ICG) (Bonnet et al. 1982), dilution volumetry cannot consistently mirror redistribution.

Study of Phentolamine Infusion

Phentolamine is a competitive α-adrenergic antagonist and has similar affinities for α_1 and α_2-receptors (Hoffman and Leftkowitz 1996). Its infusion reduces splanchnic blood perfusion (Dumont et al. 1982), inducing redistribution of blood, central hypovolemia, and peripheral blood pooling associated with a decrease in cardiac preload and afterload. Assuming that IDVG consistently measures the central ECF volume even during redistribution of blood, phentolamine infusion should produce a decrease in cardiac preload, IDVG, and CO without considerable changes in PV-ICG. We therefore designed experiments to investigate changes in IDVG and PV-ICG simultaneously before, during, and after phentolamine infusion in dogs and to test whether IDVG rather than PV-ICG has potential as an indicator of the central blood volume or central ECF volume (Matsui et al. 2000).

Fourteen mongrel dogs weighing 6.5–17.5 kg were randomly allocated into the following two groups: (1) saline group: normal saline infusion and (2) phentolamine group: phentolamine infusion 10 μg/kg min. Glucose 100 mg/kg and ICG 0.5 mg/kg were simultaneously infused through the central venous line over 30 s. Arterial blood sampling and measurement were performed in the same manner as described previously. These data served as the preinfusion values. In the phentolamine group, a bolus of phentolamine 0.1 mg/kg IV was administered followed by an infusion of 10 μg/kg min. In the saline group, the same volumes of normal saline were infused. Ninety minutes after commencing phentolamine or saline infusion, the second series of measurements were performed as previously; these data served as the during-infusion values. Phentolamine or normal saline infusion was terminated after 120 min. Ninety minutes later, the third series of measurements were conducted as previously; these data served as the postinfusion values.

An estimated blood volume (EBV) (ml/kg) was calculated as follows:

$$EBV = PV\text{-}ICG\ (ml/kg)/(1 - hematocrit(\%)/100)$$

Cardiovascular variables are shown in Table 9-1. Although pulmonary artery wedge pressure (PAWP) and central venous pressure (CVP) did not decrease either during or after the infusion in either group, CO significantly decreased during phentolamine infusion ($P < 0.05$), but not during saline infusion. During phentolamine infusion hematocrit was significantly lower than that during saline infusion ($P < 0.05$). Both total plasma protein and plasma albumin concentrations during and after the infusion decreased when compared with the corresponding preinfusion values ($P < 0.05$), but no difference was found between groups.

PV-ICG during phentolamine or saline infusion remained unchanged when compared with the corresponding preinfusion values (Table 9-2). Postinfusion PV-ICG in both groups decreased significantly when compared with corresponding preinfusion values ($P < 0.05$) reflecting that the volume of blood taken from each dog totaled approximately 40 ml for each series of measurements. IDVG significantly decreased ($P < 0.05$) during phentolamine infusion. IDVG did not change during saline infusion (Fig. 9-1; see Table 9-2), and there was a significant difference between groups ($P < 0.05$).

EBV during phentolamine or saline infusion remained unchanged when compared with the corresponding preinfusion values. Postinfusion EBV in both groups decreased significantly when compared with the corresponding preinfusion values ($P < 0.05$), but there were no differences between groups.

These results suggest a phentolamine-induced fluid shift from the central to the peripheral compartment and that an apparent overestimation of PV-ICG and EBV was unlikely, and supports the concept that IDVG, not PV-ICG, indicates the state of the central fluid volume consistently even during redistribution.

Although preinfusion CO varied markedly among dogs in either group, a linear correlation was found between IDVG and CO in the phentolamine

TABLE 9-1. Cardiovascular variables

	Saline group			Phentolamine group		
	Pre	During	Post	Pre	During	Post
Heart rate (bpm)	158 (139–198)	159 (154–183)	153 (114–190)	170 (126–207)	166 (136–207)	130 (111–183)*
Mean arterial pressure (mmHg)	130 (111–164)	145 (100–156)	145 (130–158)*	133 (98–159)	123 (102–138)	135 (81–152)
PAWP (mmHg)	10 (7–14)	13 (7–18)	14 (7–24)	8 (7–19)	9 (7–13)	10 (8–19)
CVP (mmHg)	8 (6–9)	7 (6–10)	7 (6–10)	6 (4–9)	6 (3–9)	6 (3–9)
CO (ml/kg/min)	136 (106–200)	126 (100–161)	116 (93–178)*	193 (117–227)	120 (100–192)*	100 (78–200)*
UV (ml/kg/h)	0.7 (0.1–15.4)	1.9 (0–6.3)	1.5 (0–9.8)	3.1 (0.1–11.7)	2.1 (1.6–7.6)	2.4 (0.1–2.4)
Body temperature (°C)	38.2 (36.5–39.0)	37.4 (35.1–39.0)*	36.8 (34.3–39.9)*	37.7 (36.8–38.8)	36.2 (35.0–38.0)*	34.9 (34.2–38.3)*

Values are presented as median (range)
PAWP, pulmonary artery wedge pressure; CVP, central venous pressure; CO, cardiac output; UV, urine volume; Pre, before normal saline or phentolamine infusion; During, during normal saline or phentolamine infusion; Post, 90 min after discontinuation of normal saline or phentolamine infusion
* $P < 0.05$ compared with preinfusion
Source: from Matsui et al. (2000), p 1133, table 1, with permission from Springer

TABLE 9-2. Pharmacokinetic variables

	Saline group			Phentolamine group		
	Pre	During	Post	Pre	During	Post
PV-ICG (ml/kg)	43 (35–46)	43 (33–46)	39 (34–43)*	42 (36–47)	42 (33–49)	39 (31–48)*
IDVG (ml/kg)	107 (101–122)	102 (97–120)	99.4 (90–109)*	111 (102–118)	89 (87–108)*#	93 (82–99)*#
EBV (ml/kg)	67 (61–82)	72 (61–82)	67 (55–75)*	69 (65–73)	68 (59–70)	62 (55–73)
PV-ICG/IDVG	0.39 (0.33–0.44)	0.39 (0.33–0.47)	0.40 (0.35–0.42)	0.37 (0.33–0.43)	0.46 (0.37–0.50)*#	0.42 (0.35–0.49)*
AIC for IDVG	–29.5 (–33.0 to –20.4)	–26.9 (–43.8 to –19.7)	–27.2 (–35.6 to –24.3)	–26.4 (–35.6 to –17.1)	–25.8 (–39.6 to –20.0)	–23.5 (–27.5 to –21.8)#
AIC for PV-ICG	–46.5 (–56.1 to –30.5)	–45.8 (–55.5 to –38.7)	–41.7 (–52.5 to –37.4)	–41.5 (–47.4 to –37.8)	–47.2 (–50.6 to –39.5)	–43.7 (–47.2 to –39.5)

Values are presented as median (range)
PV-ICG, plasma volume determined by indocyanine green; IDVG, initial distribution volume of glucose; EBV, estimated blood volume; Pre, before normal saline or phentolamine infusion; During, during normal saline or phentolamine infusion; Post, 90 min after discontinuation of normal saline or phentolamine infusion; AIC, Akaike's information criterion
* $P < 0.05$ compared with preinfusion; # $P < 0.05$ compared with saline group
Source: from Matsui et al. (2000), p 1134, table 3, with permission from Springer

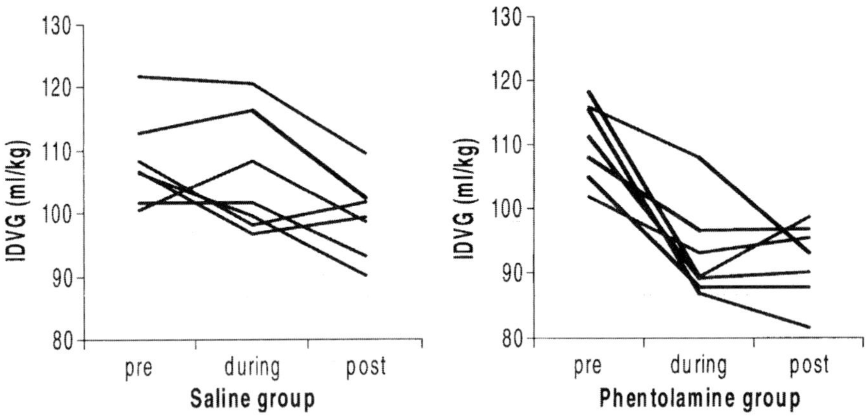

FIG. 9-1. Changes in initial distribution volume of glucose (*IDVG*) following saline or phentolamine infusion in dogs. *pre*, before normal saline or phentolamine infusion; *during*, during normal saline or phentolamine infusion; *post*, 90 min after discontinuation of normal saline or phentolamine infusion. (From Matsui et al. (2000), p 1134, fig. 1, with permission from Springer)

group ($r = 0.49$, $n = 21$, $P < 0.025$) and using all data of both groups ($r = 0.37$, $n = 42$, $P < 0.02$). However, no correlation was found between PV-ICG and CO, between CVP and CO, or between PAWP and CO using all data of either group or all data of both groups. Different pathophysiological effects other than a reduction in cardiac preload or the central blood volume may also play a role in determining CO during phentolamine infusion. For instance, a decrease in cardiac afterload would produce an increase in CO in the absence of a decrease in cardiac preload. Therefore, a correlation between IDVG and CO during phentolamine infusion in this study appears to be relatively poor compared with other IDVG studies where cardiac preload is a major determinant factor of CO, such as during a hemorrhagic experiment (Shimodate et al. 1994).

The PV-ICG/IDVG ratio during phentolamine infusion increased compared with both the corresponding preinfusion ratio and the saline group ($P < 0.05$). The postinfusion ratio in the phentolamine group tended toward preinfusion ratios but remained elevated ($P < 0.05$). The PV-ICG/IDVG ratio in the saline group remained unchanged throughout the experimental procedure.

A higher PV-ICG/IDVG ratio observed during phentolamine infusion indicates central hypovolemia and peripheral blood pooling. We also described a higher ratio as a measure of overestimation of PV-ICG in the previous chapter. In this phentolamine study, however, results did not support the presence of the overestimation. Thus, a moderately high PV-ICG/IDVG ratio (<0.50) alone would not consistently indicate the presence of leakage. As judged by the PV-ICG/IDVG ratio observed during phentolamine infusion in this study and the ratio during capillary protein leakage in our experimental animals (Sakai et al. 1998; Suzuki et al. 1999), a ratio greater than 0.50 would indicate generalized protein leakage. A ratio between 0.47 and 0.50 would indicate either possible redistribution of blood, that is, peripheral blood pooling, or leakage. In the previous chapter we proposed the threshold ratio of the overestimation was set at 0.45. However, considering the result of this experimental study, the clinically significant threshold for apparent overestimation would be 0.50, although we have not precisely tested this threshold in humans yet.

The result of this study also confirms that IDVG is not proportionally larger than the intravascular volume, and strongly supports the concept that IDVG can follow changes in the central ECF volumes, even during redistribution of fluid without gain or loss of fluid. Thus, IDVG has the potential of being an alternative measure of central blood volume or intrathoracic blood volume even during fluid shift induced by continuous infusions of vasoactive drugs.

10. IDVG and Thoracic Fluid Volume

In the previous chapter, we demonstrated that initial distribution volume of glucose (IDVG) can consistently indicate the central extracellular fluid (ECF) volume following fluid redistribution from the central to peripheral compartment. Hence, IDVG has potential as a marker for changes in cardiac preload even in the absence of fluid gain or loss. In this chapter, we evaluate the relationship between IDVG and thoracic fluid content (TFC) measured by thoracic electrical bioimpedance (TEB) in thoracic fluid-accumulated patients (Ishihara et al. 2001), and further between IDVG and intrathoracic blood volume (ITBV) (Nakamura et al. 2005; Ishihara et al. 2005b).

Thoracic Fluid Content

TEB is a noninvasive technique that analyzes changes in thoracic cavity resistance and provides cardiac output (CO) and baseline thoracic electrical bioimpedance (Z_0) across a wide range of critical conditions (Moore et al. 1991). TFC is the inverse value of Z_0, and is proportional to the thoracic fluid volume, even though a single frequency assessment cannot differentiate the site of fluid accumulation (Zarowitz and Matthie 1999). The normal value of Z_0 for adult males has been reported to be 25.0 + 5 ohms, indicating that the normal value of TFC, namely the inverse value of Z_0, ranged from 0.03 to 0.05/ohm (Pomerantz et al. 1970), or 0.034 ± 0.005/ohm for either set (Sageman 1999). Positive changes in TFC linearly reflect an increase in thoracic conductivity, which may be caused by changes in posture, loss of alveolar volume, or increases in intrathoracic fluid volume (Pomerantz et al.1970; Van De Water et al. 1973; Hemstad et al. 1994).

Clinical Study of Thoracic Fluid Accumulation

Assuming that IDVG consistently reflects the highly perfused ECF volume of the thoracic cavity, TFC and IDVG rather than TFC and indocyanine green (ICG)-derived plasma volume (PV-ICG) would move together in the same direction in thoracic fluid-accumulated patients, unless the fluid accumulates mainly in the poorly perfused part of lungs and/or the thoracic cavity, such as pleural effusion. Changes in IDVG, PV-ICG, and TFC as well as other clinical variables were simultaneously recorded in patients with or without acute thoracic fluid accumulation in the absence of apparent pleural effusion, and to test whether IDVG rather than PV-ICG reflects TFC in those patients.

ICG and glucose challenge test associated simultaneously with TEB was performed in 39 consecutive nonsurgical patients admitted to the general intensive care unit (ICU) requiring strict fluid management such as various organ failure, sepsis, pulmonary edema, congestive heart failure, and acute myocardial infarction (AMI). Eight patients were excluded from the study because of suboptimal nonevaluable bioimpedance signals or the presence of apparent pleural effusion. A total of 11 thoracic fluid-accumulated patients and 20 AMI patients were finally enrolled. The presence of apparent thoracic fluid accumulation was diagnosed from TFC by TEB > 0.05/ohm (Pomerantz et al. 1970) as well as underlying pathology. The AMI patients served as controls because none had TFC > 0.05/ohm. Although each thoracic fluid-accumulated patient might have had several determinations on different days in the ICU, only data on the day of maximal TFC and minimal TFC of this patient group were used for the study; whereas the study of the AMI patients was always performed on the day of admission to the ICU after percutaneous coronary intervention. Their cardiac symptoms had appeared within 24h before the evaluation, and 18 of the 20 AMI patients were discharged from the ICU on the subsequent morning. As part of therapy, some patients in either patient group required ventilatory support, an infusion of vasoactive drugs and/or insulin, mechanical cardiac support, and continuous hemodiafiltration.

A commercially available TEB device (Bio Z System; DynaMedic Japan, Tokyo, Japan) was attached to the patients under study. The device consists of eight skin electrodes, a laptop computer, and a software program as described previously (Clancy et al. 1991; Genoni et al. 1998). A continuous thermodilution CO monitor was attached to seven thoracic fluid-accumulated patients and all AMI patients.

Both 25 ml glucose 20% (5 g) and 10 ml ICG (25 mg) were infused simultaneously over 30 s through a central venous line or the proximal port of the pulmonary artery catheter. Arterial blood sampling and measurements were performed in the same manner as described previously.

Routine clinical variables, TFC, and pharmacokinetic variables for the thoracic fluid-accumulated patients and the AMI patients are presented in Tables 10-1 and 10-2. The incremental plasma glucose decay curve following

TABLE 10-1. Clinical variables in thoracic fluid-accumulated patients and AMI patients

	Maximal ($n = 11$)	Minimal ($n = 11$)	AMI ($n = 20$)
Incremental BW, kg	2.7 (0.6–7.5)	−0.9 (−5.9–3.0)*	0.0 (−1.6–4.3)*
Pa_{O_2}/F_{IO_2} ratio, mmHg	143 (89–315)	275 (95–395)	346 (110–546)*
Cardiac index, $l\,min^{-1}\,m^{-2}$	3.2 (2.1–5.3)	2.2 (1.6–4.5)	2.3 (1.5–4.7)
MAP, mmHg	67 (46–96)	74 (64–117)	86 (67–114)**
PAWP, mmHg	14 (9–29)	6 (3–10)**	8 (2–15)**
CVP, mmHg	10 (3–18)	3 (0–10)***	4 (0–8)*
Hct, %	27.1 (19.8–39.5)	30.9 (20.3–38.9)	39.5 (26.8–46.2)*

Values are presented as median (range)
AMI, acute myocardial infarction; maximal, thoracic fluid accumulation at maximal thoracic fluid content; minimal, thoracic fluid accumulation at minimal thoracic fluid content; incremental BW, incremental body weight above the reported basal body weight before admission to the intensive care unit; MAP, mean arterial pressure; PAWP, pulmonary artery wedge pressure; CVP, central venous pressure; Hct, hematocrit
* $P < 0.001$ vs maximal; ** $P < 0.01$ vs maximal; *** $P < 0.05$ vs maximal
Source: from Ishihara et al. Crit Care Med 2001;29:1532–1538 (p 1535, table 3), with permission from Lippincott Williams & Wilkins

TABLE 10-2. Pharmacokinetic variables in thoracic fluid-accumulated patients and AMI patients

	Maximal ($n = 11$)	Minimal ($n = 11$)	AMI ($n = 20$)
TFC	0.083 (0.055–0.1)	0.041 (0.028–0.071)*	0.038 (0.027–0.05)*
Plasma glucose (mg/100 ml)	117 (67–236)	142 (74–238)	157 (109–286)
AIC for glucose curve	−21.9 (−31.3 to −19.2)	−23.3 (−27.2 to −18.5)	−23.0 (−36.4 to −17.3)
IDVG (ml/kg)	156 (124–181)	116 (83–157)**	106 (74–135)*
Ke-gl (/min)	0.068 (0.029–0.105)	0.071 (0.041–0.094)	0.065 (0.042–0.090)
AIC for ICG curve	−43.5 (−65 to −24.1)	−44.6 (−50.4 to −29.2)	−42.9 (−54.1 to −24.9)
PV-ICG (ml/kg)	51 (44–90)	42 (27–62)***	40 (29–54)*
Ke-ICG (/min)	0.134 (0.025–0.345)	0.179 (0.021–0.418)	0.155 (0.086–0.231)
PV-ICG/IDVG ratio	0.34 (0.26–0.51)	0.36 (0.30–0.45)	0.40 (0.31–0.45)***

Values are presented as median (range)
AMI, acute myocardial infarction; maximal, thoracic fluid accumulation at maximal TFC; minimal, thoracic fluid accumulation at minimal TFC; TFC, thoracic fluid content; plasma glucose, plasma glucose present immediately before glucose challenge; AIC, Akaike's information criterion; IDVG, initial distribution volume of glucose; Ke-gl, glucose disappearance rate from plasma; PV-ICG, plasma volume determined by the indocyanine green (ICG) dilution method; Ke-ICG, ICG disappearance rate from plasma
* $P < 0.001$ vs maximal; ** $P < 0.01$ vs maximal; *** $P < 0.05$ vs maximal
Source: from Ishihara et al. (2001), p 1535, table 4, with permission from Lippincott Williams & Wilkins

glucose challenge in each thoracic fluid-accumulated patient is shown in Fig. 10-1. Central venous pressure (CVP), cardiac index (CI), and PV-ICG did not consistently move together with TFC in the same direction in each individual patient as shown in Fig. 10-2. In contrast, the incremental body weight above basal, pulmonary artery wedge pressure (PAWP), and IDVG followed the change of TFC in each patient, even though sampling size was small for PAWP measurement. TFC had a better correlation with IDVG ($r^2 = 0.41$, $P = 0.0011$, $n = 22$) than PV-ICG, CI, CVP, and the incremental body weight above basal, and inversely with either hematocrit or Pao_2/Fio_2 ratio in the

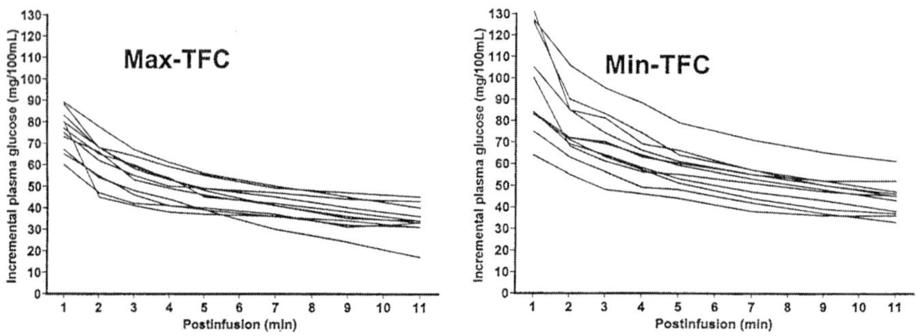

FIG. 10-1. Changes in incremental plasma glucose concentration after glucose challenge in each thoracic fluid-accumulated patient at maximal (*Max, left*) and minimal (*Min, right*) thoracic fluid content (*TFC*). (From Ishihara et al. (2001), p 1535, fig. 1, with permission from Lippincott Williams & Wilkins)

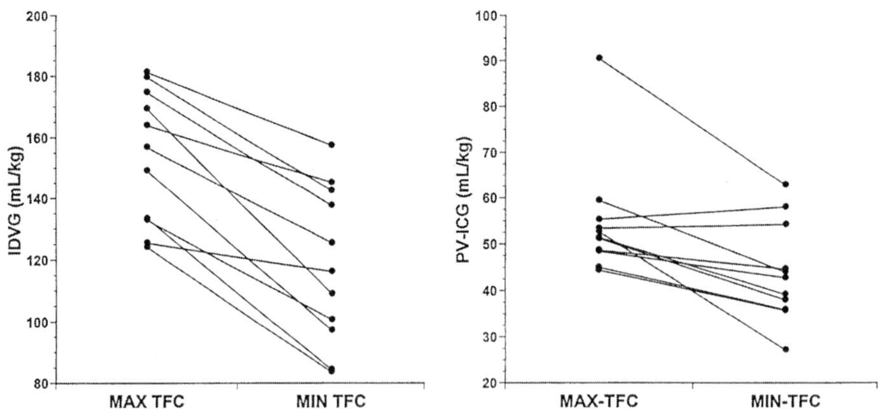

FIG. 10-2. Changes in initial distribution volume of glucose (*IDVG, left*) and plasma volume determined by indocyanine green dilution method (*PV-ICG, right*) in each apparent thoracic fluid-accumulated patient. *TFC*, thoracic fluid content; *MAX*, maximal; *MIN*, minimal. (From Ishihara et al. (2001), p 1536, fig. 2, with permission from Lippincott Williams & Wilkins)

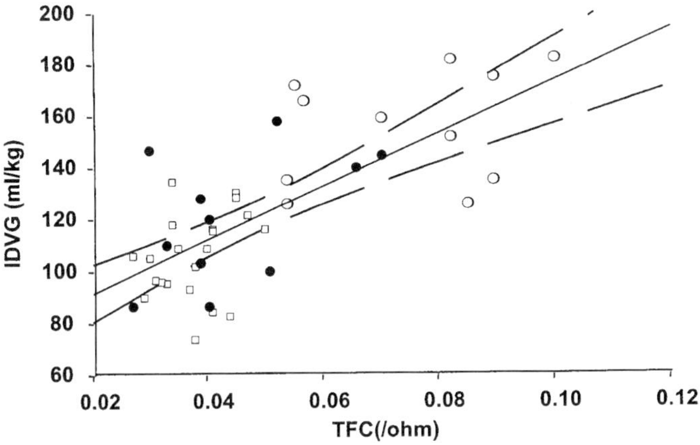

FIG. 10-3. Scatter plot for each thoracic fluid content (*TFC*) versus initial distribution volume of glucose (*IDVG*) point with or without apparent thoracic fluid accumulation. *Open and closed circles*, points at maximal and minimal TFC in thoracic fluid-accumulated patients, respectively; *squares*, points in acute myocardial infarction patients without apparent thoracic fluid accumulation; *solid line*, regression line using all data: $Y = 1000X + 71$, $r^2 = 0.52$, $P < 0.000001$; *dashed lines*, 95% confidence interval for the predicted IDVG for any given value of TFC. (From Ishihara et al. (2001), p 1536, fig. 3, with permission from Lippincott Williams & Wilkins)

thoracic fluid-accumulated patients. IDVG correlated with PV-ICG ($r^2 = 0.52$, $P < 0.001$, $n = 22$) and with CI ($r^2 = 0.29$, $P = 0.038$, $n = 14$) in those patients, respectively.

As compared with the thoracic fluid-accumulated patients at the maximal TFC, the AMI patients had normal fluid volumes as judged by the incremental body weight above basal, PAWP, CVP, IDVG, and PV-ICG (Table 10-1), There was no statistically significant correlation between TFC and other variables in the AMI patients. A linear correlation was obtained between IDVG and CI ($r^2 = 0.41$, $P = 0.0023$, $n = 20$), and between IDVG and PV-ICG ($r^2 = 0.52$, $P < 0.001$, $n = 20$) in the AMI patients.

When all data in this study were used, a linear correlation was obtained between TFC and IDVG ($r^2 = 0.52$, $n = 42$, $P < 0.001$) (Fig. 10-3) and between TFC and PV-ICG ($r^2 = 0.37$, $n = 42$, $P < 0.001$). These results suggest that IDVG has more potential than PV-ICG as an estimate of intrathoracic blood volume in critically ill patients.

Relationship Between IDVG and Thoracic Fluid Content

Results of this study demonstrated that IDVG and TFC rather than PV-ICG and TFC moved together in the same direction in each fluid-accumulated patient, and that neither PAWP, CVP, nor PV-ICG produced a better correlation with CI when compared with IDVG in patients with or without thoracic fluid accumulation.

Measurement of CO by TEB requires not only Z_0, namely the baseline value for TEB, but also other clinical variables such as arterial blood pressure. Consequently TEB is not reliable for measurement of CO in critically ill conditions, other than suboptimal nonevaluable bioimpedance signals (Moore et al. 1991; Genoni et al. 1998), whereas measurement of TFC requires Z_0 only. Presumably, TEB can be a more reliable measure for tracking TFC than CO in various critically ill conditions.

As judged by normal values of TFC described above, an apparent thoracic fluid accumulation was judged from TFC > 0.050/ohm in this study. When compared with the minimal TFC, the maximal TFC was associated with an increase in body weight above basal and corresponding increases in PAWP, CVP, IDVG, and PV-ICG. In contrast, IDVG and PV-ICG as well as TFC in the AMI patients remained normal or even low as judged by the reported normal value of IDVG and PV-ICG of 44 ± 5 ml/kg (Haller et al. 1993).

Extravascular lung water in AMI patients has been shown to correlate with PAWP (Biddle et al. 1973), but none of the AMI patients in this study had PAWP higher than 15 mmHg. This pressure monitoring supports that no obvious thoracic fluid accumulation had developed in the AMI patients, which is not surprising because deterioration of cardiac function caused by AMI would have been improved at least partly after percutaneous coronary intervention. Considering that TFC and IDVG moved together in the same direction, whereas TFC and PV-ICG did not, the former has greater potential as an alternative indicator of thoracic fluid accumulation.

In this study the thoracic fluid-accumulated patient at maximal TFC had a significantly lower PV-ICG/IDVG ratio than the AMI patients who did not have apparent thoracic fluid accumulation, indicating that the former had a relatively large IDVG associated with small PV-ICG, namely, central rather than peripheral fluid accumulation was present in those patients. A significant relationship between IDVG and CI in this study would also support the hypothesis that the former rather than PV-ICG plays a more important role in determining cardiac preload and thus, indirectly, CI.

There is a limitation in this study: the major site of fluid accumulation in the thoracic cavity cannot be identified from a single-frequency TEB alone, because changes in thoracic impedance are nonspecific, indicating only that a change has occurred in the air or fluid volume of the thoracic cavity (Van De Water et al. 1973). Not only the highly perfused extra- and intravascular volume in the thoracic cavity but also either the intracellular fluid volume or lung water in its poorly perfused part can considerably affect TFC, although none of patients in this study had apparent pleural or pericardial effusion. Indeed, 4 of 11 thoracic fluid-accumulated patients had a normal IDVG even at the maximal TFC. Thus, we cannot consistently confirm the expansion of the highly perfused ECF volume in the thoracic cavity as judged by a single-frequency TEB alone, although IDVG and TFC moved together in the same direction in the thoracic fluid-accumulated patients. In contrast, the AMI patients had normal TFC without an apparent increase in body weight above basal, which corresponds with a report that consistent changes in bioelectrical impedance require body weight changes greater than 3 kg (Roos et al. 1993). These findings would allow speculation that TFC is not sensitive enough as an indicator of the intrathoracic blood volume or the intrathoracic highly perfused ECF volume. Additionally, some patients cannot be evaluated because of suboptimal bioimpedance signals. Thus, TFC alone should not be used as an indicator of the cardiac preload.

Intrathoracic Blood Volume Measured by Single Transpulmonary Technique

Measurement of intrathoracic blood volume (ITBV) has become clinically possible as a more sensitive measure of cardiac preload than cardiac filling pressures (Lichtwarck-Aschoff et al. 1992; Gödje et al. 2000; Boussat et al. 2002). ITBV consists of global end-diastolic volume (GEDV), pulmonary blood volume, and part of the aortic blood volume, depending on the position of the recording catheter (Hedenstierna 1992). GEDV consists of the sum of the end-diastolic volumes of all four chambers of the heart. ITBV is basically calculated as the product of cardiac output (CO) and the mean transit time (MTT) of the indicator between the site of injection and the site of the detection (Sakka et al. 2000a) (Fig. 10-4). Originally, the double-indicator technique was introduced for ITBV measurement (Lichtwarck-Aschoff et al. 1992; Hoeft et al. 1994), and recently the single transpulmonary technique was also introduced (Buhre et al. 1998). The two measurement methods proved to be identical in humans (Buhre et al. 1998; Neumann 1999; Sakka et al. 2000). Inaccuracy of ITBV measurement has been reported in the presence of aortic aneurysm, cardiac diseases, intracardiac shunts, pulmonary perfusion abnormalities (Sakka et al. 2000a), and reduced left ventricular function (Mundigler et al. 2000).

Accuracy of Cardiac Output Using the Single Transpulmonary Dilution Technique

The reported bias between CO using the single transpulmonary dilution technique and CO using a Swan–Ganz catheter was -0.04 ± 0.41 l/min during

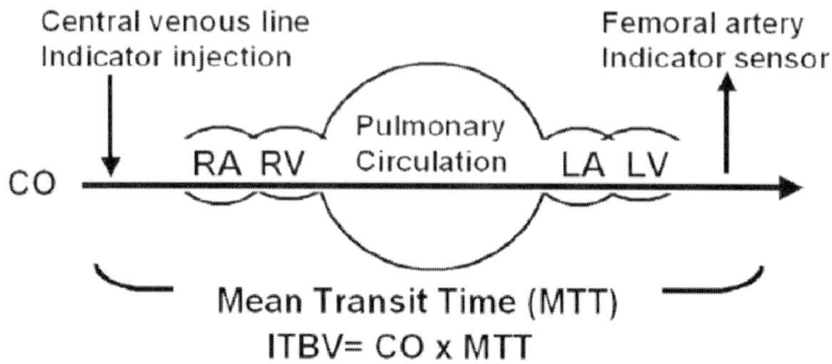

FIG. 10-4. Principle of intrathoracic blood volume (ITBV) measurement. CO, cardiac output; RA, right atrium; RV, right ventricle; LA, left atrium; LV, left ventricle; MTT, mean transit time; ITBV, intrathoracic blood volume

experimental hypovolemia and fluid resuscitation in dogs (Friedman et al. 2002). In the clinical setting, a close agreement between these two intermittent CO measurements has also been observed during lung transplantation (Della Rocca et al. 2002) or during off-pump coronary artery bypass grafting (Gödje et al. 1999), even though a close agreement between these two measurements has not been consistently observed during cardiac surgery using hypothermic cardiopulmonary bypass (Rauch et al. 2002). Accordingly, CO measurement using the PiCCO system appears to be reliable similar as that using a Swan Ganz catheter, unless there is apparent cardiac pathology.

Normal ITBV Value

Preisman et al. (1997) reported ITBV using the thermo-dye dilution technique in dogs. Blood loss and volume loading in their study was similar to that in our experimental study (Nakamura et al. 2005). Their normovolemic ITBV value was 31.5 ± 5.5 ml/kg; the ITBV value after 30% blood volume loss was 24.5 ± 5.0 ml/kg, and the value after volume loading was 35.2 ± 7.0 ml/kg. Each of these values is comparable with the corresponding values of our experiment, suggesting that either technique can equivalently measure ITBV even in dogs. The reported normal indexed ITBV (ITBVI) in mechanically ventilated patients ranged from 800 to 1000 ml/m^2 (Lichtwarck-Aschoff et al. 1992). Reported ITBVI at the end of surgery for lung transplantation ranged from 458 to 1206 ml/m^2 (Della Rocca et al. 2002).

Experimental Study of Hemorrhagic Hypotension and Subsequent Volume Loading

Fourteen mongrel dogs were used for the study. A flexible 4-Fr. catheter with an integrated thermistor (Pulsiocath PV2014L13; Pulsion Medical Systems, Munich, Germany) was inserted into the left femoral artery to determine CO and ITBV using the single indicator technique. The catheter was connected to the measurement device (model PiCCO; Pulsion Medical Systems) to measure ITBV. A flow-directed pulmonary arterial catheter was also inserted. Before each glucose and ICG administration, CO and ITBV were measured using 5 ml chilled 0.9% saline solution. Subsequently, both glucose 100 mg/kg and ICG 0.5 mg/kg were injected simultaneously through the external jugular vein within 4 s to measure IDVG and ICG-derived plasma volume (PV-ICG). Arterial blood sampling and measurement were performed in the same manner as described in the previous chapters. Ninety minutes after the end of the first series of measurements, blood was withdrawn at 1 ml/kg min over 30 min. Thirty minutes after completion of hypovolemia, the second series of measurements and blood sampling were performed. Ninety minutes after the end of the second series of measurements, 90 ml/kg lactated Ringer's solution was given over 30 min, followed by the third series of measurements and blood sampling.

Changes in cardiovascular variables are shown in Table 10-3. IDVG decreased during hypovolemia ($P < 0.001$) and increased after volume loading

TABLE 10-3. Changes in cardiovascular and associated measurements

	Normovolemia	Hypovolemia	Volume loading
Cardiac output ($ml\,kg^{-1}$)	181 ± 51	93 ± 34**	188 ± 62##
Heart rate (bpm)	181 ± 23	183 ± 31*	154 ± 31#
Mean arterial pressure (mmHg)	139 ± 16	105 ± 35**	127 ± 15
Mean pulmonary arterial pressure (mmHg)	19 ± 4	15 ± 4	24 ± 8##
Mean pulmonary capillary wedge pressure (mmHg)	11 ± 3	9 ± 3	13 ± 3#
CVP (mmHg)	7.6 ± 1.2	4.6 ± 1.9**	7.6 ± 1.5##
Hematocrit (%)	41.2 ± 5.5	35.2 ± 3.8*	23.9 ± 6.4#
Plasma total protein concentration ($g\,dl^{-1}$)	4.9 ± 0.5	3.9 ± 0.6**	2.6 ± 0.5**##
Arterial blood temperature (°C)	38.0 ± 1.2	37.7 ± 1.7	36.0 ± 2.3*

Data are given as mean ± SD
* $P < 0.05$ vs normovolemia; ** $P < 0.01$ vs normovolemia; # $P < 0.05$ vs hypovolemia; ## $P < 0.01$ vs hypovolemia
Source: from Nakamura et al. (2005), p 204, table 1

compared with hypovolemia ($P < 0.001$) (Table 10-4). PV-ICG decreased during hypovolemia ($P = 0.001$) and increased after volume loading compared with hypovolemia ($P < 0.001$). ITBV decreased during hypovolemia ($P = 0.002$) and increased after volume loading compared with hypovolemia ($P < 0.001$).

Linear correlations were obtained between IDVG and ITBV ($r^2 = 0.52$, $n = 42$, $P < 0.001$) (Fig. 10-5) and between IDVG and CO ($r^2 = 0.56$, $n = 42$, $P < 0.001$). Linear correlations were also observed between changes in IDVG (ΔIDVG) and those in ITBV (ΔITBV) ($r^2 = 0.76$, $n = 28$, $P < 0.001$) (Fig. 10-6a), and between ΔIDVG and changes in CO (ΔCO) ($r^2 = 0.81$, $n = 28$, $P < 0.001$) (Fig. 10-6b). The ITBV/IDVG ratio during normovolemia was 0.26 ± 0.04, which remained unchanged throughout the procedure. We conclude that

TABLE 10-4. Changes in fluid volumes

	Normovolemia	Hypovolemia	Volume loading
IDVG ($ml\,kg^{-1}$)	113 ± 15	85 ± 17*	123 ± 20**
Plasma glucose ($mmol\,l^{-1}$)[a]	6.0 ± 0.8	5.8 ± 1.4	5.5 ± 1.0
PV-ICG ($ml\,kg^{-1}$)	46 ± 7	36 ± 5*	50 ± 8**
ITBV ($ml\,kg^{-1}$)	29 ± 4	22 ± 5*	33 ± 7**
ITBV/IDVG ratio	0.26 ± 0.04	0.26 ± 0.04	0.26 ± 0.05

Data are expressed as mean ± SD
[a] Plasma glucose concentration present before glucose injection
* $P < 0.01$ vs normovolemia; ** $P < 0.01$ vs hypovolemia
Source: from Nakamura et al. (2005), p 204, table 2

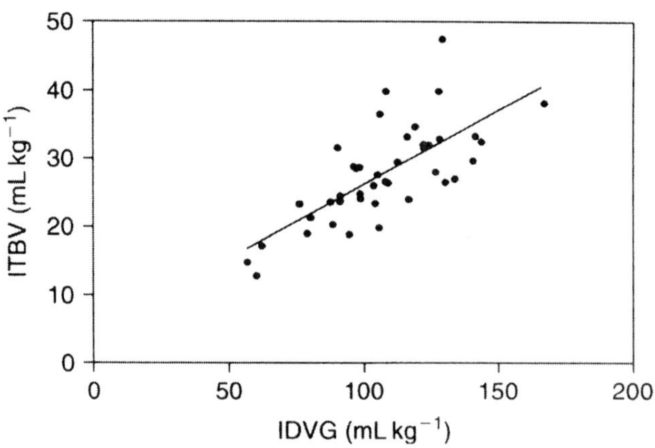

FIG. 10-5. Relationship between IDVG and ITBV. The *straight line* is the regression line ($Y = 0.2X + 4.4$, $r^2 = 0.52$, $P < 0.001$). (From Nakamura et al. (2005), p 205, fig. 1, with permission from Cambridge University Press)

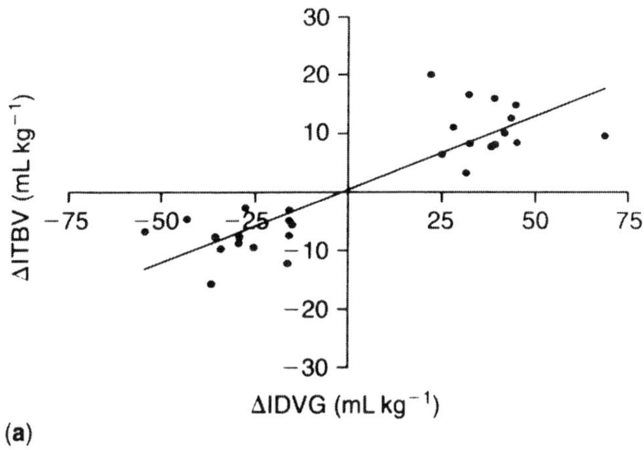

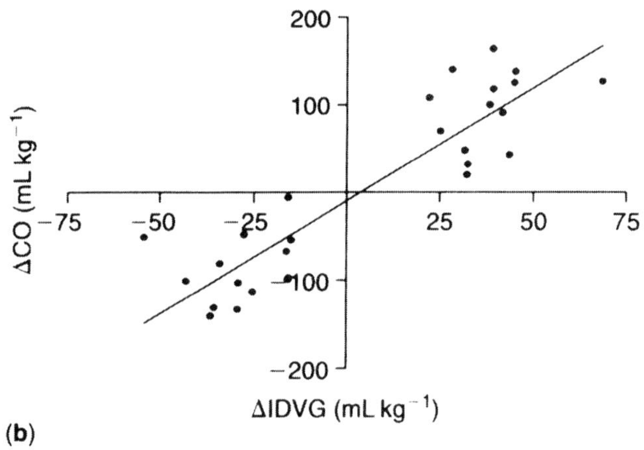

FIG. 10-6. Regression analysis between changed variables. **a** Change in IDVG versus change in ITBV. Linear correlation was observed ($r^2 = 0.76$, $P < 0.001$). **b** Change in IDVG versus change in cardiac output. Linear correlation was observed ($r^2 = 0.81$, $P < 0.001$). ΔIDVG, change in IDVG; ΔITBV, change in ITBV; ΔCO, change in cardiac output. (From Nakamura et al. (2005), p 205, fig. 2, with permission from Cambridge University Press)

IDVG has a linear correlation with ITBV in experimental hypovolemia and subsequent volume loading.

Clinical Study of Hypovolemic Hypotension and Subsequent Volume Loading

In the foregoing experimental study, a considerable time was allowed before each measurement after a relatively stable hemodynamic state had been achieved following experimental interventions. Thus, it remains unclear whether IDVG can consistently follow acute hemodynamic changes in critical conditions. Seventeen consecutive surgical patients admitted postoperatively to the intensive care unit (ICU) were initially enrolled into the study. Twelve of these patients who developed hypovolemic hypotension during the first 10h postoperative were enrolled into the study. Preoperative echocardiographic examination revealed that left ventricular ejection fraction was higher than 60% in each patient. Each patient underwent radical surgery for esophageal cancer performed through a right thoracoabdominal approach along with extensive resection of adjacent lymph nodes, subcarinal lymph nodes, and/or cervical lymph nodes, and stayed in the ICU for at least the first 2 postoperative days. Neither vasoactive drugs nor blood products were administered when patients arrived at the ICU. All patients postoperatively received mechanical ventilatory support at least until the first postoperative morning. Both 4.3% glucose solution with electrolytes and lactated Ringer's solution were infused simultaneously at a constant rate of 1.5 ml/kgh for the former and 1.0 ml/kgh for the latter throughout at least 12h after surgery. No vasoactive drugs were administered throughout the study period. One patient required a continuous infusion of insulin (1 U/h) throughout the study period.

Hypovolemic hypotension was defined as follows. Volume loading was clinically required when either of the following conditions was met during the first postoperative 10h: (1) systolic arterial blood pressure <90 mmHg lasting longer than 5 min without an increase in CVP, or (2) a reduction of arterial blood pressure >40 mmHg compared with the value immediately after admission to the ICU lasting longer than 5 min without an increase in CVP.

Measurements were made three times: immediately after admission to the ICU on the operative day, during clinically defined hypotension, and 10 min after completion of volume loading with 250 ml 10% low molecular weight dextran over 20–30 min. A right subclavian venous catheter had been placed before the operative day. A thermistor-tipped catheter for thermodilution and pulse contour analysis (PV2015L13; Pulsion) was inserted into a femoral artery and connected to the PiCCO monitoring system (Pulsion) in the ICU immediately after surgery as has been described elsewhere (Sakka et al. 2000a). Then, 10 ml cold isotonic saline solution (<8°C) was injected through the right subclavian venous line to determine ITBV. Immediately after measurement of ITBV, CO, and routine cardiovascular variables, 10 ml 50% glucose solution (5 g) was injected through the same central venous line to calculate IDVG. Blood samples were obtained through a radial artery catheter immediately before and at 3, 4, 5, and 7 min after injection.

A minimal postoperative bloody drainage on the operative day and a relatively stable cardiovascular state on the first postoperative day without

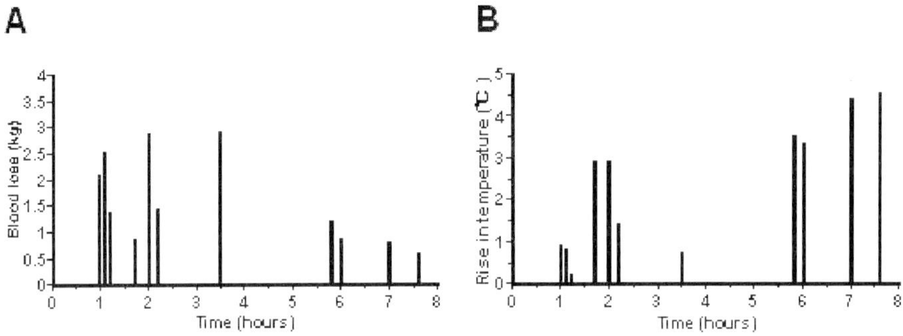

FIG. 10-7. Relationship between estimated intraoperative blood loss and time difference between hypotension and the first measurement (**A**), and between an increase in blood temperature when hypotension developed compared with admission to the intensive care unit (ICU) and time difference between hypotension and the first measurement (**B**). *Time*, time difference between hypotension and the first measurement. (From Ishihara et al. (2005b), p 1715, fig. 1, with permission from *Chest*)

requiring blood transfusion did not support the presence of apparent continued hemorrhage in this study. Hypotension associated with an increase in heart rate occurred at an average of 3.4 ± 2.5 h, ranging from 1 h to 7.6 h after the first measurement. Six patients whose hypotension occurred during the first 4 h had estimated intraoperative blood loss greater than 1000 g (Fig. 10-7A) and five of them received both packed red cells and colloidal solutions in the operative room, whereas three patients whose hypotension occurred thereafter had intraoperative blood loss less than 1000 g, and one of them received colloidal solutions in the operating room.

In all patients, the peripheral skin was cold on admission to the ICU, and thereafter became warm associated with an apparent increase in blood temperature, particularly in the late study period (see Fig. 10-7B). Hypotension occurred during the first 4 h and was associated with a decrease in cardiac index (CI) in seven of eight patients. Hypotension occurred thereafter was associated with an increase in CI in three of four patients as compared with the first measurement (Fig. 10-8). Table 10-5 shows cardiovascular variables and fluid volumes in three sets of measurements. When hypotension developed, CVP, indexed ITBV (ITBVI), and stroke volume index were decreased ($P < 0.01$, respectively), but both indexed IDVG (IDVGI) and CI remained statistically unchanged, even though these five values were increased after volume loading compared with hypotension ($P < 0.001$, respectively).

Actual IDVGI correlated only slightly with actual ITBVI ($r^2 = 0.23$, $n = 36$, $P = 0.003$), even though a moderate correlation was observed as the two volumes changed ($r^2 = 0.69$, $n = 24$, $P < 0.001$) (Fig. 10-9). Actual IDVGI also

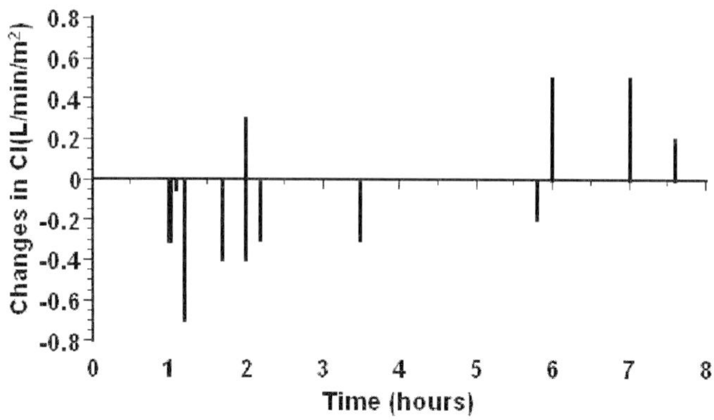

Fig. 10-8. Changes in cardiac index (*CI*) when hypotension developed compared with the first measurement immediately after admission to the ICU in each individual patient. *Time*, time difference between hypotension and the first measurement. (From Ishihara et al. (2005b), p 1716, fig. 2, with permission from *Chest*)

correlated only slightly with actual SVI ($r^2 = 0.39$, $n = 36$, $P < 0.001$), even though a moderate linear correlation was observed as the two volumes changed ($r^2 = 0.72$, $n = 24$, $P < 0.001$) (Fig. 10-10A,B). Either actual or changed IDVGI correlated moderately with that of CI ($r^2 = 0.61$, $n = 36$, $P < 0.001$; $r^2 = 0.82$, N = 24, $P < 0.001$) (Fig. 10-10C,D). Either actual or changed ITBVI correlated moderately with that of SVI ($r^2 = 0.56$, $n = 36$, $P < 0.001$; $r^2 = 0.82$, $n = 24$, $P < 0.001$). Actual ITBVI correlated only slightly with actual CI ($r^2 = 0.32$, $n = 36$, $P < 0.001$), even though a moderate correlation was observed between these two changed values ($r^2 = 0.69$, $n = 24$, $P < 0.001$). We conclude that IDVGI cannot equivalently be used as an alternative measure of ITBVI or SVI during hemodynamically unstable states after esophagectomy.

Relationship Between IDVG and ITBV

Our experimental results support the concept that measurement of IDVG can follow changes in ITBV in the various fluid volume states. Gabbanelli et al. (2004) also demonstrated a moderate linear correlation between IDVGI and ITBVI in critically ill patients without capillary protein leakage ($r^2 = 0.79$). They also showed a good ability of IDVG to reflect cardiac index variations by using receiver operating characteristic curve analysis (Fig. 10-11). However, our clinical study after esophagectomy demonstrates that IDVGI is correlated only slightly with ITBVI in the three sets of measurement. As judged by clinical conditions including amounts of intraoperative blood loss

Table 10-5. Cardiovascular variables and fluid volumes

	ICU admission	Hypotension	Volume loading
Heart rate (bpm)	78 ± 17 (50–120)	92 ± 17 (75–125)*	85 ± 14 (58–106)#
SAP (mmHg)	122 ± 28 (87–174)	88 ± 9 (76–109)***	105 ± 16 (82–139)*##
MAP (mmHg)	90 ± 19 (64–121)	63 ± 8 (50–76)***	72 ± 10 (53–91)***
CI ($l/min/m^2$)	2.6 ± 0.4 (2.0–3.4)	2.5 ± 0.5 (1.8–3.7)	3.5 ± 0.5 (2.9–4.6)***###
SVI (ml/m^2)	35 ± 9 (17–48)	29 ± 8 (21–44)**	42 ± 9 (31–60)**###
CVP (mmHg)	8 ± 2 (4–12)	7 ± 3 (2–12)**	9 ± 3 (5–15)**###
Hematocrit (%)	30.9 ± 4.6 (24.3–39.1)	31.2 ± 5.0 (24.9–41.8)	25.9 ± 4.3 (20.4–34.9)***###
Plasma glucose (mmol/l)	8.3 ± 1.4 (5.6–10.1)	8.1 ± 1.8 (5.3–11.0)	8.7 ± 1.9 (5.8–11.7)
IDVGI (l/m^2)	3.6 ± 0.4 (3.1–4.2)	3.4 ± 0.5 (2.7–4.3)	4.1 ± 0.5 (3.4–4.8)***###
ITBVI (l/m^2)	0.90 ± 0.1 (0.67–1.12)	0.81 ± 0.15 (0.61–1.14)**	0.95 ± 0.14 (0.75–1.17)###

Data are presented as mean ± SD (range)

SAP, systolic arterial pressure; MAP, mean arterial pressure; CI, cardiac index; SVI, stroke volume index; CVP, central venous pressure; plasma glucose, plasma glucose levels immediately before glucose injection; IDVGI, indexed initial distribution volume of glucose; ITBVI, indexed intrathoracic blood volume

* $P < 0.05$, ** $P < 0.01$, and *** $P < 0.001$ compared with immediately after ICU admission, respectively; # $P < 0.05$, ## $P < 0.01$, and ### $P < 0.001$ compared with during hypotension, respectively

Source: from Ishihara et al. (2005b), p 1716, table 2, with permission from *Chest*

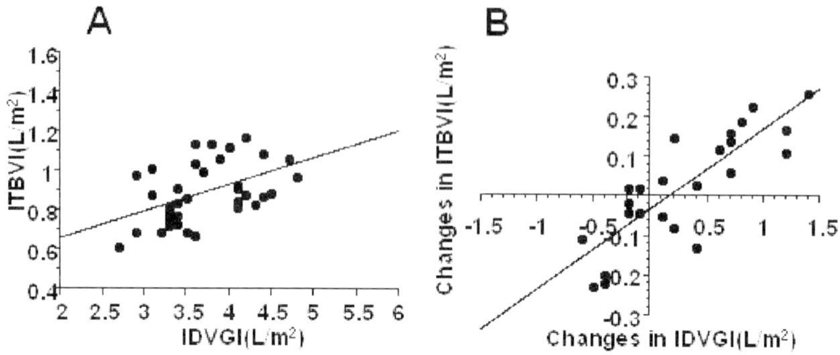

FIG. 10-9A,B. Relationship between indexed initial distribution volume of glucose (*IDVGI*) and indexed intrathoracic blood volume (*ITBVI*). **A** Actual values: $Y = 0.14X + 0.38$, $r^2 = 0.23$, $n = 36$, $P = 0.003$; **B** changed values: $Y = 0.2X - 0.035$, $r^2 = 0.69$, $n = 24$, $P < 0.0001$. (From Ishihara et al. (2005b), p 1717, fig. 4, with permission from *Chest*)

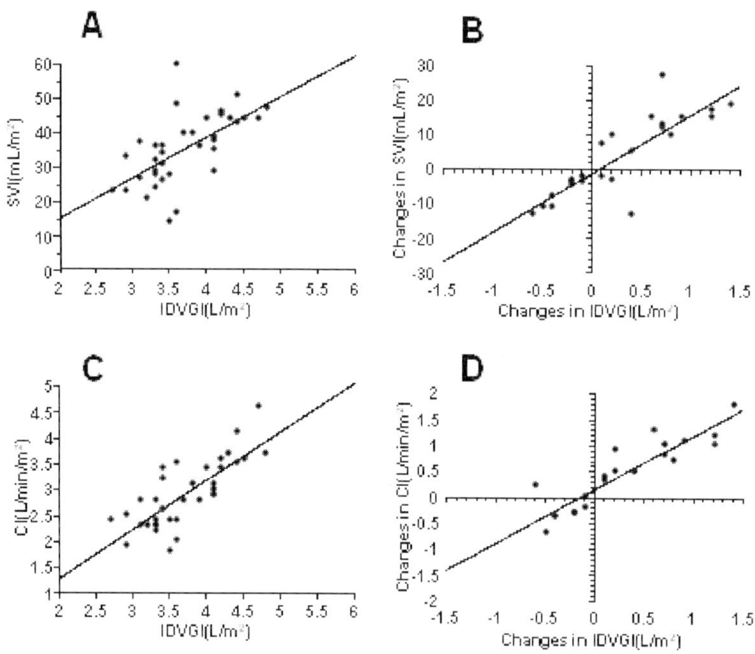

FIG. 10-10A–D. Relationship between indexed initial distribution volume of glucose (*IDVGI*), stroke volume index (*SVI*), and cardiac index (*CI*). **A** Actual values between IDVGI and SVI: $Y = 12X - 8.3$, $r^2 = 0.39$, $n = 36$, $P < 0.001$; **B** changed values between IDVG and SVI: $Y = 17X - 1.3$, $r^2 = 0.72$, $n = 24$, $P < 0.001$; **C** actual values between IDVGI and CI: $Y = 0.94X - 0.59$, $r^2 = 0.61$, $n = 36$, $P < 0.001$; **D** changed values between IDVGI and CI: $Y = X + 0.14$, $r^2 = 0.82$, $n = 24$, $P < 0.001$. From (Ishihara et al. (2005b), p 1718, fig. 5, with permission from *Chest*)

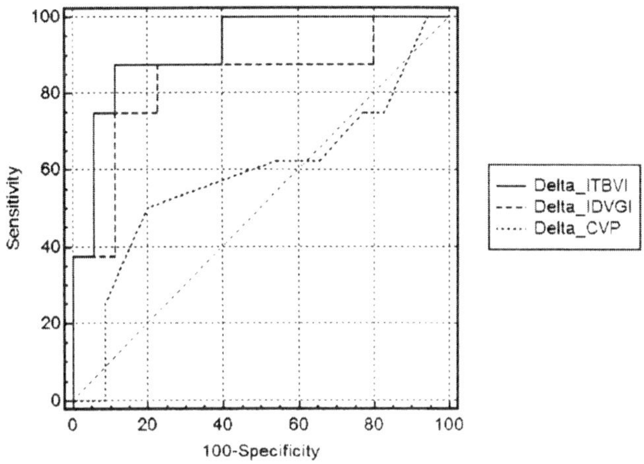

FIG. 10-11. Receiver operating characteristic (ROC) curve analysis comparing variations in ΔITBVI, ΔIDVGI, Δ central venous pressure (ΔCVP), and CI. ΔCI of at least 0.1 was considered a positive change. The areas under the ROC curve were ΔITBVI 0.92 (confidence interval, 0.80–0.97), ΔIDVGI 0.82 (confidence interval, 0.69–0.91), and CVP 0.58 (confidence interval, 0.44–0.72). (From Gabbanelli et al. (2004), p 2071, fig. 3, with permission from Springer)

and peripheral circulatory state when hypotension developed, hypotension during the first 4h of the study period may be mainly attributable to hypovolemia, even though neither arterial blood pressure nor blood lactate levels immediately after admission to the ICU indicated the presence of apparent oxygen deficit in the peripheral tissues at that time, whereas hypotension thereafter may be mainly attributable to the redistribution of blood from the central to the peripheral tissues, as judged by improved peripheral circulation.

A simultaneous decrease in CVP, ITBVI, SVI, and CI in this study would support a decrease in cardiac preload or hypovolemic hypotension, whereas a decrease in CVP, ITBVI, and SVI, but not CI, would support a simultaneous decrease in cardiac preload and afterload. Changes in heart rate and systemic inflammatory response syndrome after esophagectomy (Nakanishi et al. 2000) would also play a role in determining CI, at least partly. Presumably, there may be several contributory factors to affect CI in each individual patient of this study.

In contrast to ITBVI, neither CI nor IDVGI was consistently decreased when hypotension developed. However, the relationship between IDVGI and CI in this study ($r^2 = 0.61$) was comparable with that of our previous daily-based studies after esophagectomy ($r^2 = 0.50$) (Ishihara et al. 2000c) and early after major burn ($r^2 = 0.69$) (Ishihara et al. 1998a). We also observed a linear correlation between IDVG and CO after an infusion of phentolamine that yields fluid redistribution from the central to the peripheral compartment (Matsui et al. 2000). Furthermore, 22 plots of 24 changes in IDVGI and CI moved together to the same direction in this study, as shown in Fig. 10-10D. These findings would allow speculation that the IDVGI–CI relationship is consistent even during hypotension.

Considering capillary membrane permeability of glucose (Guyton and Hall 2000a), glucose can rapidly distribute throughout the central ECF compartment even in a low CO state; this is supported by the fact that a relatively large IDVG was observed even in the presence of a small CO in patients with congestive heart failure (Ishihara et al. 1996a). Accordingly, IDVG may be variable depending on the size of the central ECF volume with minimal effects of CO states. As IDVG is apparently greater than ITBV, IDVG would reflect not only cardiac preload or ITBV, but also rapidly exchanging extravascular fluid volume or the central ECF volume. Nevertheless, a good correlation has been consistently observed between IDVG and CO in critically ill patients without congestive heart failure, as described in Chapter 6.

Considering the result of this study, IDVG measurement cannot be equally used as a measure of cardiac preload. However, it may be of benefit in decision making even immediately after hypotension has developed whether volume loading or administration of vasopressors is required for treatment, because IDVGI has a closer correlation with CI as compared with either ITBVI or SVI in this study. Although we gave fluid volume loading to all patients when hypotension developed in this study, it would have been more appropriate to give vasoactive drugs such as norepinephrine instead of fluid volume loading in some patients associated with an increase in IDVGI or CI.

11. Indirect Measurement of Red Cell Volume

Anemia is a commonly observed problem in the intensive care unit (ICU). Hematocrit (Hct) or hemoglobin levels have been used empirically to decide when to transfuse erythrocytes despite the fact that single Hct or hemoglobin measurements may not be reliable for this purpose in ICU patients (Marino 1997). Measurement of red cell volume (RCV) would help provide more reliable information for transfusion purposes because volume loading or fluid restriction is commonly performed in the ICU. However RCV indicators, even those using a nonradioactive tracer such as sodium fluorescein, generally require labeling of the patient's erythrocytes, blood sampling, and subsequent measurement of blood tracer concentration (Orth et al. 1998).

These complicated procedures would limit the utility of such RCV measurement in the ICU. In contrast, indocyanine green (ICG) has been used as an indicator of plasma volume (PV-ICG). This technique does not require labeling and can be repeatedly performed at 30-min intervals provided hepatic function is normal (Haruna et al. 1998). Although Busse and colleagues (1993) reported that comparative measurements of blood volume using ICG and ^{51}Cr-labeled red cells differed by only 1.7% in neurosurgical ICU patients, our institution does not permit the use of radioisotopic markers for the estimation of intravascular volume. Thus, an alternative approach is required to test the accuracy of intravascular volume measurements. Assuming that RCV [calculated from PV-ICG and arterial Hct (RCV-ICG)] is an index of erythrocyte volume, it follows that this should remain unchanged, regardless of changes in either arterial PV-ICG or Hct, provided there is no gain or loss of erythrocytes. To our knowledge, no previous studies have been performed to evaluate the repeatability of RCV-ICG measurements. As volume loading or fluid restriction is usually required in critically ill patients during the early period following ICU admission, daily changes in either PV-ICG or arterial Hct are likely to occur.

Indirect Measurement of RCV

We retrospectively evaluated the repeatability of RCV-ICG measurements in nonsurgical cardiac or respiratory patients without clinical evidence of blood gain or loss on the first 2 successive ICU days. A combined ICG and glucose challenge test was performed daily in 121 consecutive critically ill nonsurgical cardiac or respiratory patients admitted to the ICU requiring strict fluid management. Although each patient had undergone several daily fluid volume determinations during their ICU stay, only two successive measurements performed on the first and second ICU days were used in this analysis. A medical student (Sachiko Tsukamoto), who was blinded to fluid volume measurement results, reviewed each patient's ICU records to determine whether there was evidence of blood loss or erythrocyte transfusion between the two measurements. Internal blood loss includes gastrointestinal or tracheobronchial bleeding, cardiac tamponade, and hematoma formation. In addition, external bleeding from vascular access sites, blood loss from extracorporeal circuits, bloody drainage, and blood sampling >50 ml/day were also checked. Fifty of 121 patients were judged to have neither blood gain nor loss between measurements and were initially included in the study. Eight of 50 patients had possible overestimation of PV-ICG as judged by an PV-ICG/IDVG ratio greater than 0.45 on either study day, resulting in possible inaccuracy of RCV-ICG determination as described in Chapter 8. Consequently, these eight patients were also excluded from the study. The remaining 42 patients with the following main diagnoses—acute myocardial infarction (AMI) after percutaneous coronary intervention ($n = 20$), congestive heart failure ($n = 6$), and acute respiratory failure ($n = 16$)—were finally included for analysis.

As part of therapy, 24 patients required mechanical ventilation, 23 patients required an infusion of vasoactive drugs such as epinephrine, norepinephrine, dobutamine, and dopamine, 16 patients required an infusion of insulin ranging from 0.5 to 5.0 units/h, 17 patients required intraaortic balloon pumping, and 8 patients required continuous hemodiafiltration on either study day. Continuous thermodilution cardiac output (CO) (Vigilance Monitor, model VGSSYS; Baxter, Irvine, CA, USA) was monitored in 37 patients.

ICG 25 mg in 10 ml glucose 50% (5 g) solution was administered as a single bolus injection through a central venous catheter as described previously. The coefficient of variation for repeated measurements of Hct (range, 16%–55%) was 1.5% or less. Arterial Hct and other routine clinical variables were recorded immediately before each ICG and glucose challenge. RCV-ICG was then calculated from PV-ICG and arterial Hct (%) as follows:

RCV-ICG = PV-ICG × 0.01 Hct/(1 − 0.01 Hct)

Body weight was measured immediately after admission to the ICU and subsequently on the second ICU day at 8:30 A.M.

Daily body weight and routine cardiovascular variables remained unchanged (Table 11-1). PV-ICG on the second day increased when compared with the first day by an average of 0.17 l ($P = 0.004$) associated with a decrease in Hct by an average of 2.0% ($P < 0.001$) (Table 11-2). RCV-ICG decreased on the second day by an average of 0.02 l ($P = 0.038$), whereas IDVG was unchanged. The bias of repeated measurements of RCV-ICG was −0.02 ± 0.06 l, or −1.8% ± 5.1% (Fig. 11-1).

There were eight patients whose CO was low (<2.5 l/min/m^2) in one of the two measurements. The lowest CO was 1.4 l/min/m^2. The bias of RCV-ICG measurement in these patients was −0.02 ± 0.04 l. In addition, seven patients had a low ICG plasma disappearance rate (Ke-ICG) (<0.10/min) in both measurements, with the lowest Ke-ICG being 0.014/min. The daily bias of RCV-ICG in these patients was −0.02 ± 0.04 l. Only one patient had both a low and a normal Ke-ICG value on two study days (0.085/min and 0.136/min, respectively). The daily RCV-ICG difference in this patient was 0.02 l. We conclude that RCV-ICG is useful for the evaluation of daily RCV status provided there is no overestimation of PV-ICG.

TABLE 11-1. Routine cardiovascular variables and therapeutic supports

	First day	Second day
Body weight (kg)[a]	58.4 ± 10.3 (38.6–82.6)	58.3 ± 10.4 (38.7–82.9)
Heart rate (beats/min)	98 ± 22 (47–138)	94 ± 16 (67–144)
MABP (mmHg)	74 ± 15 (5–109)	78 ± 15 (50–110)
CVP (mmHg)	6 ± 4 (0–15)	6 ± 5 (0–19)
Cardiac index (l/min m^2)	2.8 ± 1.0 (1.5–7.1)	3.1 ± 0.8 (1.9–4.6)
Ventilatory support	24	21
Vasoactive drugs	22	23
Insulin	16	16
IABP	16	17
CHDF	8	6

Values are presented as mean ± SD (range)

MABP, mean artery blood pressure; CVP, central venous pressure; Ventilatory support, number of patients who required mechanical ventilatory support; Vasoactive drugs, number of patients who required an infusion of vasoactive drugs such as dopamine, dobutamine, norepinephrine, or epinephrine; IABP, number of patients who required cardiac support with an intraaortic balloon pump; CHDF, number of patients who required continuous hemodiafiltration; Insulin, number of patients who required an infusion of insulin

[a] Body weight was measured immediately after admission to the intensive care unit (ICU) and at 8:30 A.M. on the 2nd ICU day

TABLE 11-2. Fluid volumes on the first and the second days

	First day	Second day	P
Hematocrit (%)	31.2 ± 6.9 (20.1–50.3)	29.2 ± 5.4 (20.4–38.5)	<0.001
PV-ICG (l)	2.60 ± 0.50 (1.52–3.54)	2.77 ± 0.48 (1.99–3.82)	$P = 0.004$
Ke-ICG (/min)	0.155 ± 0.079 (0.020–0.423)	0.169 ± 0.079 (0.014–0.439)	NS
RCV-ICG (l)	1.19 ± 0.40 (0.67–2.21)	1.17 ± 0.40 (0.62–2.16)	$P = 0.038$
RCV-ICG (ml/kg)[a]	20.5 ± 5.2 (11.6–31.8)	20.2 ± 5.4 (11.0–31.8)	NS
Plasma glucose (mg/100 ml)	172 ± 73 (36–339)	144 ± 45 (34–242)	$P = 0.043$
IDVG (l)	7.05 ± 1.37 (3.50–9.36)	7.32 ± 1.50 (3.50–10.2)	NS
Ke-glucose (/min)	0.073 ± 0.017 (0.040–0.110)	0.065 ± 0.016 (0.037–0.096)	$P = 0.004$
PV-ICG/IDVG ratio	0.37 ± 0.04 (0.28–0.45)	0.38 ± 0.04 (0.29–0.44)	NS

Values are presented as mean ± SD (range)
PV-ICG, plasma volume determined by the indocyanine green (ICG) dilution method; Ke-ICG, ICG disappearance rate from plasma; RCV-ICG, red cell volume calculated from PV-ICG and arterial hematocrit; Plasma glucose, plasma glucose levels present before glucose challenge; IDVG, initial distribution volume of glucose; Ke-glucose, glucose disappearance rate from plasma
[a]RCV-ICG based on the reported basal body weight before admission to the intensive care unit

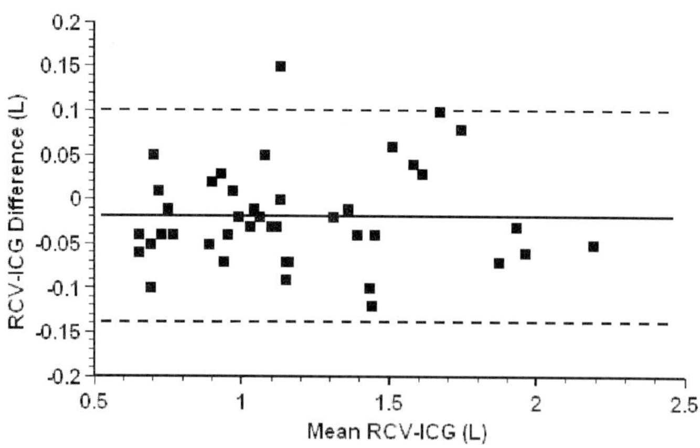

FIG. 11-1. Daily differences of red cell volume calculated from indocyanine green-derived plasma volume and arterial hematocrit (RCV-ICG) according to Bland and Altman's method. *Solid* and *dashed lines* represent mean and 95% confidence limits, respectively

Repeatability of Indirect Measurement of RCV

In several reports, reliability or repeatability of PV-ICG measurement was tested at a short time interval in the absence of changes of fluid volume (Busse et al. 1993; Haller et al. 1993; Jones and Wardrop 2000). However, no reports using the ICG dilution method, including noninvasive pulse dye densitometry, have focused on the repeatability of RCV measurements. Although the presence of unrecognized hemorrhage could not be completely ruled out and the total volume of daily blood sampling for routine clinical examination and for the purposes of this study was approximately 30 ml, the repeatability of RCV-ICG (−1.8% ± 5.1%) would be comparable with the reported bias of PV-ICG measurements (−1.3% ± 4.3%) (Haller et al. 1993).

Normal RCV is 30 ± 5 ml/kg in men and postmenopausal women and 25 ± 5 ml/kg in younger women (Jones and Wardrop 2000). Busse and colleagues (1993) reported that comparative measurements of blood volume using ICG or ^{51}Cr-labeled red cells differed by only 1.7% in neurosurgical ICU patients. Mean RCV-ICG and Hct values on both study days in this study were approximately 20 ml/kg and 30%, respectively. Although the accuracy of each individual RCV-ICG calculation requires direct measurement of RCV, these findings would allow speculation that an erroneously large overestimation of RCV-ICG is unlikely in this study.

There were some patients who had either a low cardiac output or a low Ke-ICG in this study. However, we have previously reported that a low cardiac output (<2.5 l/min m^2) or a low Ke-ICG (<0.1/min) does not significantly affect the result of PV-ICG measurements (Ishihara et al. 1999). As judged by the small bias of RCV-ICG in these patients, these critical conditions would not produce a significant error in RCV-ICG.

Rehm et al. (2001) observed a larger mean PV-ICG (1700–1750 ml/m^2) after induction of anesthesia but before surgery when compared with normal plasma volume (1395 ± 349 ml/m^2) (Pearson et al. 1995). They also reported a large discrepancy between arterial Hct and whole-body Hct, where whole-body Hct was calculated from RCV (detected using sodium fluorescein) and PV-ICG. We (Mi et al. 2003) found that PV-ICG after induction of anesthesia was also increased by around 11% when compared with an increase in plasma volume calculated from the dilution of arterial Hb and Hct following induction. Considering any possible overestimation of PV-ICG and then RCV-ICG, simultaneous measurement of IDVG would help evaluate the accuracy of PV-ICG measurement. Based on results of Chapters 8 and 9, a PV-ICG/IDVG ratio higher than 0.50 would indicate apparent overestimation, a ratio ranging from 0.45 to 0.50 would indicate either possible overestimation or redistribution of fluid from the central to peripheral compartment, and a ratio less than 0.45 would indicate accurate measurement.

Based on the results of this study, an increase in PV-ICG observed on the second study day would also support a hemodilutional reduction of Hct on that day. Accordingly, Hct alone would not consistently indicate RCV status in each nonsurgical critically ill patient even where there was no blood gain or loss soon after admission to the ICU. Furthermore, approximately 60% of patients who were initially enrolled into the study had some bleeding problems. Thus, daily RCV measurement is desirable to evaluate whether RCV loss occurs in critically ill patients. However, dilution volumetry generally requires tedious blood sampling and is time consuming, which would limit routine clinical application of this method. Noninvasive ICG pulse dye densitometry (DDG analyzer; Nihon-Kodan, Tokyo, Japan) and glucose measurement (Diasensor; Diasense, Pittsburgh, PA, USA) have become clinically possible, even though the currently available technologies would not reliably measure either concentration in critically ill patients. These advanced technologies may have a significant impact on both fluid and blood transfusion management in the near future.

12. IDVG and Prediction of Hypovolemic Hypotension

Major surgery induces a significant shift of the extracellular fluid (ECF) from the central to the peripheral compartment that occurs intraoperatively and lasts postoperatively (Gold 1992). The central ECF consists of the interstitial fluid (ISF) in highly perfused organs such as heart, lungs, kidneys, and liver as well as plasma, and the peripheral ECF consists of the ISF in less-perfused organs such as muscle, fat, and subcutaneous tissues. In Japan, a radical operation for esophageal carcinoma including three-field lymph node (cervical, thoracic, and abdominal lymph nodes) dissection has been extensively performed. After surgical procedure, therefore, lymph flow from these areas is not able to enter the systemic circulation, at least partly.

This surgical procedure consistently produces great surgical stress as compared with other surgical procedures (Fig. 12-1). Postoperative apparent cardiovascular instability is very common, and frequent hypotensive episodes are observed throughout the first 48h postoperatively. According to our experience, more than 60% of patients who underwent radical surgery for esophageal carcinoma developed hypovolemic hypotension postoperatively on the operative day, even though operative hemorrhage and/or postoperative bloody drainage were minimal and hemodynamic states immediately after surgery were stable. Presumably, the postoperative hypovolemic hypotension would be a result of a further reduction in the central ECF volume.

Routine hemodynamic variables such as cardiac output (CO), central venous pressure (CVP), and pulmonary artery wedge pressure are commonly used to evaluate the intravascular volume or cardiac preload. Intraoperative fluid balance study is also used for assessment of intravascular volume immediately after surgery. However, none of these measures reliably indicates the intravascular volume status (Shippy et al. 1984). Thus, an alternative simple and rapid measure is crucial to assess the intravascular volume or cardiac preload.

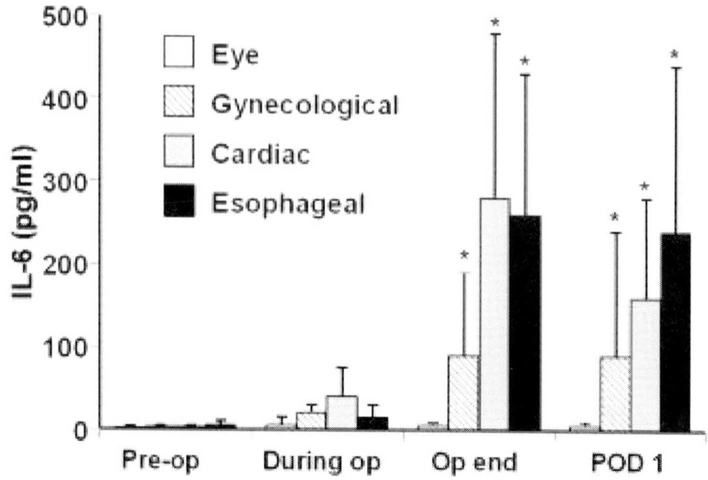

FIG. 12-1. Plasma interleukin (IL)-6 concentrations following various surgical procedures following total intravenous anesthesia with propofol, ketamine, and fentanyl. Data are presented as mean (SD). *Op*, operation; *POD 1*, First postoperative day. *, $p < 0.05$ vs. Pre-op. (From Hashimoto and Ishihara (1997), p 84, fig. 2; with permission from Kokuseidoh)

Study of Hypovolemic Hypotension After Esophagectomy

Assuming that initial distribution volume of glucose (IDVG) rather than routine cardiovascular variables consistently mirrors the state of the central ECF volume or cardiac preload, IDVG has potential as an alternative indicator of fluid management. We examined which variables immediately after surgery can predict subsequent hypovolemic hypotension through the first 15h after radical surgery for esophageal cancer (Suzuki et al. 2001).

Twenty-five consecutive patients who were admitted to our intensive care unit (ICU) immediately after radical surgery for esophageal cancer were studied (Table 12-1). Intraoperative fluid management was determined by each anesthesiologist who did not know the contents of this study. All patients postoperatively remain intubated and received mechanical ventilatory support by 10 cmH_2O of pressure support without applying positive end-expiratory pressure. No infusion of vasoactive drugs such as dopamine and dobutamine was given during the study. A 4.3% glucose solution with electrolytes was infused at a constant rate of 2 ml/kgh throughout the first postoperative day. Intraoperative fluid balance was calculated as a simple sum of infused crystalloids and colloids, minus urine and estimated blood loss. Immediately after admission to the ICU, both 25 ml 20% glucose (5 g)

TABLE 12-1. Characteristics of patients

	Median (range)
Number (male/female)	25 (24/1)
Age (years)	63 (44–76)
Body weight (kg)	54.9 (40.0–80.0)
Operation time (min)	520 (270–806)
Fluid in (ml)	3600 (2200–8000)
Blood loss (g)	473 (150–1720)
Urine (ml)	658 (211–1230)

Fluid in, intraoperatively administered fluid volume; blood loss, estimated intraoperative blood loss
Source: from Suzuki et al. (2001), p 1149, table 1, with permission from Lippincott Williams & Wilkins

and 10 ml indocyanine green (ICG) (25 mg) were infused over 30 s through the central venous line. Blood samplings and measurements were performed in the same manner as described previously.

During the first 15 h postoperatively, hypovolemic hypotension was diagnosed as follows: systolic arterial blood pressure (ABP) either 70–80 mmHg lasting longer than 30 minutes or less than 70 mmHg at any time, accompanied by either tachycardia (heart rate >120/min) or oliguria (urine volume <10 ml/h), and responsive to IV fluid administration (lactated Ringer's solution 500–1000 ml or colloid 250–500 ml). Hematocrit (Hct) and ICG-derived plasma volume (PV-ICG) were measured again 15 h later as performed previously, to compare values including the circulating blood volume (= PV-ICG/(1 – Hct/100)) with those on admission to the ICU. Postoperative drainage volumes were also measured.

Intraoperatively, neither hypotension nor tachycardia was observed. Eight patients underwent hemodilutional autologous blood transfusion of 350–860 ml, and six patients were given plasma protein fraction of 250–1000 ml. Neither packed red cell nor fresh-frozen plasma was given intraoperatively and during the first 15 h postoperatively.

The median IDVG and PV-ICG on admission to the ICU were 104 ml/kg for the former and 47 ml/kg for the latter. A significant relationship was observed between IDVG and PV-ICG ($r = 0.65$, $n = 25$, $P < 0.001$). IDVG correlated well with CO ($r = 0.89$, $n = 25$, $P < 0.001$). Although PV-ICG also had a linear correlation with CO ($r = 0.58$, $n = 25$, $P = 0.003$), the correlation was less than that of IDVG and CO ($P < 0.001$).

Although no patient had episodes of systolic ABP less than 75 mmHg, 11 patients met the criteria of subsequent hypovolemic hypotension. Furthermore, 5 patients developed hypotension at least twice after initial treatment that required more intravenous fluid administration. Either lactated Ringer's solution (500–1000 ml) or plasma protein fraction (250–500 ml) was administered as needed. Ten of 14 patients whose IDVG was less than 105 ml/kg and 11 of 15 patients whose cardiac index (CI) was less than 3.4 l/min m^2 required additional IV fluids to overcome hypotension, and a statistical difference was observed with or without hypovolemic hypotension ($P < 0.001$, respectively) (Fig. 12-2). None of the other measures correlated with clinical hypovolemia (Fig. 12-2). Plasma glucose decay curves after glucose infusion of each patient in the two groups with or without hypovolemic hypotension are shown in Fig. 12-3. The 95% confidence limits of IDVG with or without hypovolemic hypotension ranged from 87 to 102 ml/kg for the former or from 105 to 133 ml/kg for the latter. When the cutoff of IDVG for prediction of hypovolemic hypotension was set at 105 ml/kg, sensitivity of prediction was 71% and specificity was 91%.

The median Hct immediately after surgery was 36.2% in the patients with hypovolemic hypotension and 32.6% in those without hypotension. There was no significant difference in Hct with or without hypovolemic hypotension. The median circulating blood volumes immediately after admission to

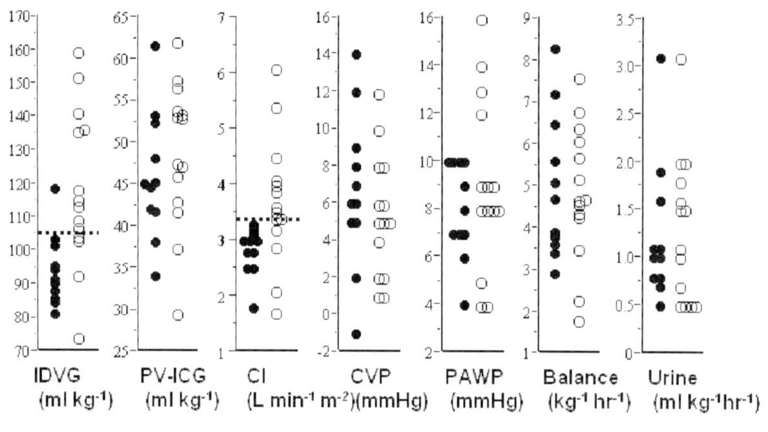

Fig. 12-2. Comparison between each clinical variable and hypovolemic hypotension. *IDVG*, initial distribution volume of glucose; *PV-ICG*, plasma volume determined by the indocyanine green dilution method; *CI*, thermodilution cardiac index; *CVP*, central venous pressure; *PAWP*, pulmonary artery wedge pressure (each measured on admission to the intensive care unit); *Balance*, simple sum of intraoperative fluid balance study; *Urine*, intraoperative urine volume. *Open circles* indicate patients who did not develop subsequent hypovolemic hypotension through the first 15 h postoperatively; *closed circles* indicate patients associated with subsequent hypovolemic hypotension; *dashed lines* in the IDVG and CI columns are dividing lines with or without hypovolemic hypotension (105 ml/kg, $P = 0.002$, for the former; 3.4 l min^{-1} m^{-2}, $P = 0.0003$ for the latter). (From Suzuki et al. (2001), p 1149, fig. 3, with permission from Lippincott Williams & Wilkins)

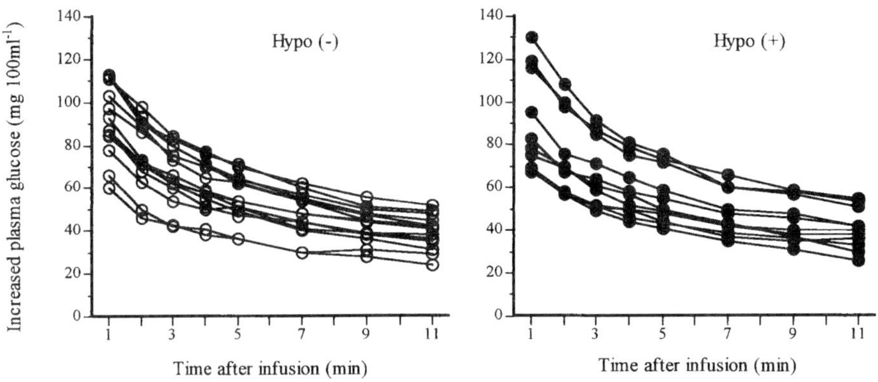

FIG. 12-3. Plasma glucose decay curves after IV infusion in each patient in the two groups with or without subsequent hypovolemic hypotension. *Hypo (–)*, patients who did not develop subsequent hypovolemic hypotension throughout the first 15h postoperatively; *Hypo (+)*, patients associated with subsequent hypovolemic hypotension. (From Suzuki et al. (2001), p 1150, fig. 4, with permission from Lippincott Williams & Wilkins)

the ICU were 68 (48–90) ml/kg in the hypovolemic patients and 76 (49–84) ml/kg in the patients without hypovolemia, even though no significant difference developed between the patient groups. The circulating blood volumes remained statistically unchanged after 15h [61 (54–83) ml/kg for the former and 68 (57–86) ml/kg for the latter, respectively] compared with volumes immediately after admission to the ICU, even though hypovolemia was transiently treated. Postoperative drainage volumes during the first 15h were similar in both groups. Results suggest that IDVG can help predict the subsequent hypovolemic hypotension early after radical surgery for esophageal cancer.

Relationship Between IDVG and Subsequent Hypovolemic Hypotension

When hypotension occurs in the early postoperative period, postoperative hemorrhage should be initially considered, even though many other factors may be responsible. However, we believe apparent postoperative hemorrhage did not account for the hypotension in this study, because Hct and calculated circulating blood volumes on the first postoperative morning remained unchanged as compared with the first measurement of this study. Furthermore, postoperative acute cardiac failure was unlikely because each hypotensive episode was responsive to intravenous fluid administration.

IDVG and CO had a moderate linear correlation in this study as observed previously, and either IDVG or CO could predict subsequent hypotension, even though PV-ICG could not predict it and correlated less with CO. The critical IDVG for hypovolemic hypotension was 105 ml/kg, which is relatively low as compared with normal IDVG, approximately between 110 and 130 ml/kg, as described in Chapter 4. However, we were not able to perform IDVG measurements during the subsequent hypotension, which occurred mostly during the night after surgery. After this study we also measured IDVG and CO during subsequent hypotension after esophagectomy (Ishihara et al. 2005b). Interestingly, in some patients whose hypotension developed during the later period of the operative day, both IDVG and CO remained unchanged or even increased despite hypotension. Thus, both IDVG and CO early after surgery cannot consistently predict hypovolemic hypotension that occurred during the later period of the operative day (after 6h or more). Further detailed discussion on this subject is available in Chapter 10. Additionally, IDVG measurement cannot reliably predict subsequent hypotension after cardiac surgery (Harvey et al. 2003), because this surgical procedure is frequently associated with internal bleeding, temperature change, alterations in vasomotor tone and myocardial contractility, and/or fluid shifts during the early postoperative period (Ishihara 2006).

Although severe hypovolemia can be detected by routine cardiovascular variables, a smaller volume depletion or overload cannot consistently be detected even when a flow-directed pulmonary artery catheter is used, as observed in this study. Accordingly, inadequate blood flow in several important organs such as the gastrointestinal tract can occur despite these variables being normal. However, the magnitude of perioperative fluid shifts would vary widely among patients, even if the surgical procedure were standardized.

Results of this study support the fact that IDVG is useful as an indicator of the central ECF volume status or cardiac preload. In addition, it is useful as a guide for early postoperative fluid management, even though the critical volume of subsequent hypovolemic hypotension may vary depending on surgical procedures and the underlying pathology of each patient. At least daily measurement of IDVG is recommended for decision making in daily fluid management in critically ill patients.

13. Case Presentation

Case 1. Acute Adrenal Insufficiency Early After Major Vascular Surgery

We had a patient who developed severe hypotension shortly after aortic surgery (Ishihara et al. 1996b). We could not convincingly rule out the presence of hypovolemia in this patient. Consequently, we performed initial distribution volume of glucose (IDVG) measurement, and the result showed that obvious hypovolemia was not present. In retrospect, the patient was found to have developed acute adrenal insufficiency at that time.

A 67-year-old man (basal preoperative body weight, 51.5 kg) was admitted to the ICU immediately after emergency operative repair of a ruptured abdominal aortic aneurysm. The patient was hypothermic. Two hours later, when normal body temperature had been restored with the aid of a forced-air warming blanket, the patient became hypotensive: arterial blood pressure (ABP) of 78/40 mmHg was associated with mean central venous pressure (CVP) of 0 mmHg and heart rate of 120/min (Table 13-1). These variables were corrected by infusions of 1000 ml blood and 560 ml colloidal solution over 2 h. However, at 6 h after ICU admission, ABP again started to decrease gradually, and at 10 h, it fell to 82/52 mmHg associated with CVP of 4 mmHg and heart rate of 112/min. During this 10-h period the patient became agitated and frequently complained of abdominal and back pain. A total of 0.6 mg buprenorphine was administered. Bloody drainage continued consistently at a rate of approximately 30 g/h. Postoperative hemorrhage was strongly suspected to be the major cause of the hypotension, and a further 400 ml blood and 500 ml lactated Ringer's solution were administered rapidly, associated with a postoperative routine crystalloid infusion (90 ml/h).

However, 11 h after ICU admission, his blood pressure had deteriorated, although radial pulsation was easily palpable and his skin was warm. Analysis of arterial blood gases with Fio_2 0.4 by face mask had revealed pH

TABLE 13-1. Sequential changes in hemodynamic parameters after admission to the ICU

Time (h)	0	2	4	6	8	10	11
ABP (mmHg)	125/68	78/40	106/60	110/66	90/48	82/52	55/30
CVP (mmHg)	2	0	7	3	4	4	7
HR (bpm)	122	120	106	110	112	112	122
BE ($mEq \cdot l^{-1}$)	–7.4	—	–1.6	–1.0	—	–4.0	–5.0
Hb ($g \cdot 100\,ml^{-1}$)	7.8	—	8.5	9.5	—	9.5	10.0
UV ($ml \cdot h^{-1}$)	34	32	100	150	12	12	0
BT (°C)	34.4	36.3	37.7	37.7	37.9	38.2	38.0
Rapid administration							
Blood (ml)		1000				400	
Colloid (ml)		560				—	
Lactated Ringer's solution (ml)		—				500	

ICU, intensive care unit; ABP, arterial blood pressure; CVP, central venous pressure; HR, heart rate; BE, base excess; Hb, hemoglobin; UV, urine volume; BT, body temperature
Source: from Ishihara et al. (1996b), p 70, table 1, with permission from Springer

7.41, Pa_{CO_2} 30 mmHg, Pa_{O_2} 67 mmHg, and base excess –4.0 mEq/l. Laboratory values included white blood cell count 10 000/mm^3, hemoglobin 10.0 g/100 ml, serum sodium 127 mEq/l, serum potassium 4.8 mEq/l, serum chloride 105 mEq/l, serum lactate 5.5 mmol/l, and blood urea nitrogen 35 mg/100 ml. We then decided to measure IDVG. An infusion of 25 ml glucose 20% (5 g) was administered over 30 s, and arterial blood samples were drawn before the infusion and at 3, 4, 5, and 7 min postinfusion. Plasma glucose concentration was 76 mg/100 ml before the challenge and 130, 123, 119, and 113 mg/100 ml at 3, 4, 5, and 7 min postinfusion, respectively. Computed IDVG was 7.22 l (140 ml/kg) and approximated IDVG was 7.45 l (145 ml/kg), which indicated that the patient was not hypovolemic. In addition, abdominal ultrasonography did not reveal any hemorrhage. Thus, we believed that cardiovascular collapse in the absence of hypovolemia had developed in this patient. At that time, neither a total of 40 mg IV ephedrine nor an infusion of dobutamine up to 15 μg/kg min improved his situation.

Subsequently, an infusion of epinephrine was started at 0.1 μg/kg min and increased up to 0.7 μg/kg min without a significant heart rate change. In the meantime, investigation of this patient's medical history revealed he had been taking 5 mg prednisone daily for 15 years because of polymyositis. Acute adrenal insufficiency was immediately suspected, and an IV bolus of 1 g methylprednisolone was given. Immediately after the injection, ABP increased to 138/62 mmHg, associated with resolution of the patient's agitated mental status. Consequently, the infusion of epinephrine was tapered off and discontinued at 2 h after the methylprednisolone injection. Thereafter, the patient had a relatively uneventful postoperative course, received glucocorticoid coverage, and required no further rapid blood or fluid infusions during his ICU stay. He was discharged from the ICU on the 4th postoperative day. However, the patient suddenly died of unknown causes on the 16th postoperative day. Autopsy revealed marked bilateral atrophy of the adrenal glands.

In retrospect, the plasma cortisol level immediately before the methylprednisolone injection was 20.5 μg/100 ml, which indicated that the hypothalamic–pituitary–adrenal axis could not adequately respond to acute stress in this patient (normal range, >22 μg/100 ml during acute stress (Passmore 1985).

Comments

This event occurred during the relatively early years after we started to measure IDVG in the ICU. At that time, echocardiography was not routinely available in our ICU. In retrospect, we should have measured IDVG immediately on admission to the ICU or during the first hypotensive episode using the simple approximation method.

Case 2. Postoperative Continued Bloody Drainage Associated with Hypotension

According to our experience, cardiac surgical patients often develop postoperative hypotension early after admission to the ICU, and this may even occur in those patients who are receiving infusions of vasoactive drugs. We had a postcardiac surgical patient whose cardiac filling pressures kept decreasing in the early postoperative period, whereas the IDVG remained elevated or normal even during hypotension. In retrospect, IDVG seems to be more reliable as an indirect cardiac preload as compared with cardiac filling pressures.

A 71-year-old man (basal preoperative body weight, 68 kg; height, 169 cm) was admitted to the ICU following aortic valve replacement and replacement of the ascending aorta. He had been receiving an infusion of dobutamine 2 μg/kg min from the operating room. A relatively large amount of bloody drainage had continued postoperatively in the operating room, even though it decreased gradually after admission to the ICU. Thus, we decided to keep the patient on a ventilator by using an infusion of propofol so long as bloody drainage continued. One hour after the admission, his ABP became 140/50 mmHg, associated with heart rate 76/min, cardiac output (CO) 7.2 l/min, pulmonary artery wedge pressure (PAWP) 10 mmHg, CVP 9 mmHg, and hemoglobin concentration in blood 8.3 g/100 ml. IDVG at that time was 10.0 l (147 ml/kg). Amount of hourly drainage was 270 ml. Two hours later, hourly bloody drainage decreased to 105 ml. However, his ABP was 76/38 mmHg, heart rate 66/min, CO 4.9 l/min, PAWP 9 mmHg, and CVP 4 mmHg. His hemoglobin concentration in blood was 8.1 g/100 ml and IDVG was 8.3 l (122 ml/kg).

The surgeons requested that we give a blood transfusion to this patient. However, normal IDVG value and high urine output of 150 ml/h without use of diuretics as well as a gradual decrease in bloody drainage at that time did not support hypovolemia. Consequently, we did not give any blood transfusion to this patient, but we decided to discontinue the infusion of propofol, because his respiratory data had not deteriorated after surgery, and his trachea was then extubated. After discontinuation of propofol, his ABP returned to 110/50 mmHg, associated with heart rate 68/min, CO 4.6 l/min, CVP 3 mmHg, PAWP 4 mmHg, and IDVG 8.1 l (119 ml/kg). The patient was discharged on the first postoperative morning in satisfactory condition without any further blood transfusion or increased infusion rate of vasoactive drugs.

Comments

This case showed that IDVG is useful even in postcardiac surgical patients for decision making about blood transfusion or an increase in the infusion rate of vasoactive drugs. CO after cardiac surgery varied, obviously reflecting not only cardiac preload but also cardiac contractility, cardiac afterload, and heart rate. Thus, it is very difficult to assess cardiac preload from routine cardiovascular variables during hemodynamically unstable states. In this patient, IDVG remained elevated or normal even during considerable variability of CO. Presumably, a propofol infusion that induced a decrease in either cardiac afterload or cardiac contractility may have had a major impact on decreased CO and hypotension in this patient.

Case 3. Postoperative Hypotension Associated with Limited Cardiac Function

We had a cardiac surgical patient with limited cardiac reserve associated with possible continued postoperative internal bleeding. This case could confirm the usefulness of IDVG measurement in limited cardiac reserve.

A 74-year-old man (preoperative basal body weight, 52 kg; body surface area, 1.52 m^2) was admitted to the ICU immediately after emergency repair of ventricular septal perforation. Intraaortic balloon pumping (IABP) was started from the operating room in response to limited left ventricular function. On arrival to the ICU, infusion of norepinephrine 0.1 μg/kg min was discontinued because of a transient rise of ABP up to 160/90 mmHg, but thereafter ABP and CO decreased to 70/40 mmHg and 2.8 l/min, respectively (Table 13-2). Approximated IDVG at that time was 5.9 l (113 ml/kg), indicating normal, but with a relatively small central fluid volume despite minimal bloody drainage. Accordingly, colloidal solution of 500 ml was rapidly given, and an infusion of norepinephrine 0.2 μg/kg min was restarted. Although cardiac filling pressures increased significantly, ABP and CO remained low, suggesting that poor cardiac contractility played a major role in the continued low CO state of this patient, despite cardiac preload being normal or even augmented. An additional infusion of dobutamine 1 μg/kg min was subsequently started. CO, ABP, and urine volume increased significantly during the next 4 h. However, CO, ABP, and cardiac filling pressures again decreased on the first postoperative morning.

Hypovolemia was strongly suspected. However, the result of approximated IDVG determination at that time (7.8 l, 150 ml/kg) did not support the presence of hypovolemia, but rather indicated increased central ECF volume. Thus, no further volume loading was planned. During the first postoperative

TABLE 13-2. Sequential changes in hemodynamic variables after admission to the ICU

Time	Admission 02:00	POD0 02:30	POD0[a] 03:00	POD1 06:57	POD1 13:00	POD2 09:30	POD2 17:00	POD3 13:00
Body weight (kg)	52.9			53.1		52.4		49.9
IDVG (l)	5.9			7.8	7.7	9	7	8.1
IDVG (ml/kg)	113			150	148	173	135	155
Cardiac output (l/min)	2.9	3	4.2	3.4	3.2	4.2	4.2	3.8
Cardiac index (l/min m^2)	1.86	1.92	2.7	2.2	2.1	2.7	2.7	2.4
Systolic ABP (mmHg)	83	70	100	84	84	116	123	126
Mean ABP (mmHg)	58	50	75	62	56	79	84	89
PAWP (mmHg)	8	8	10	8		6	6	4
CVP (mmHg)	8	7	11	6	5	4	3	3
Noradrenaline (μg/kg min)			0.2	0.2	0.2	0.2	0.2	0.2
Dobutamine (μg/kg min)			1	1	1	2	2	2
IABP	1:1	1:1	1:1	1:1	1:1	1:1	1:1	1:1
Urine volume (ml/h)	350	80	160	70	55	130	170	155

Admission, immediately after admission to the ICU; POD, postoperative day; ABP, arterial blood pressure; PAWP, pulmonary artery wedge pressure; CVP, central venous pressure; IABP, intraaortic balloon pumping

[a] After start of an infusion of dobutamine (1 μg/kg min) following negligible effects of volume loading with plasma protein fraction and low molecular weight dextran

afternoon, CO and ABP remained low, associated with decreased cardiac filling pressures. However, proximal IDVG remained elevated (7.71, 148 ml/kg). Infusion rate of dobutamine was increased to 2 μg/kg min. Thereafter, CO became improved, and good spontaneous urinary flow was observed (>100 ml/h). On the second postoperative morning, body weight decreased associated with a stable hemodynamic state. The patient was discharged thereafter.

Comments

This case would also support the view that changes in cardiac filling pressures do not consistently indicate that cardiac preload and IDVG rather than cardiac filling pressures is more useful and reliable for decision making about therapeutic interventions. Additionally, repeated IDVG measurement is useful, and it can be done even during a low CO state, as described in Chapter 6.

Case 4. Pulmonary Embolism Associated with Right Ventricular Dysfunction

We had a patient with pulmonary embolism associated with right ventricular dysfunction. This underlying pathology could affect the IDVG measurement as an indirect measure of cardiac preload.

An 86-year-old woman (reported basal body weight, 56 kg) was referred from an affiliated hospital to our ICU due to pulmonary embolism. Her Pao_2 was 72 mmHg with oxygen mask (Fio_2, 0.4). Echocardiographic examination revealed apparent enlargement of the right ventricle associated with shift of the ventricular septum toward the left ventricule. Her ABP and CVP were 100/60 mmHg and 19 mmHg, respectively. IDVG immediately after admission to the ICU was 4.83 l (86 ml/kg), indicating that the central ECF volume was obviously low despite the increased size of the right ventricle.

For this patient, we gave fluid volume loading without an additional infusion of vasoactive drugs to overcome hypotension according to the findings of the IDVG study. The patient's cardiovascular state became stable even in the presence of pulmonary embolism.

Comments

This case would confirm that IDVG measurement cannot detect the specific volume change of each cardiac chamber but rather mirrors the central ECF fluid volume as a whole. Therefore, when anatomical abnormality of cardiac chambers is present, as described in this case, caution should be used in the interpretation of the results of the IDVG measurement. Further studies are required for therapeutic decision making in such patients.

Case 5. Inadequate Echocardiographic Assessment

We had a patient who developed hypotension immediately after admission postoperatively to the ICU. Echocardiographic examination revealed that the left atrium and ventricle were relatively small in size at that time. In contrast, both IDVG and PV-ICG were large enough to maintain CO.

A 76-year-old man (preoperative basal body weight, 43 kg; height, 160 cm) was admitted to the ICU after emergency colostomy and bowel resection for acute perforation with peritonitis. A large amount of norepinephrine infusion had been started from the operating room due to septic shock associated with acute renal failure. On arrival at the ICU, his ABP was 79/36 mmHg and CVP 3 mmHg, associated with sinus tachycardia 110/min, despite continuous infusions of both norepinephrine 0.2 μg/kg min and dobutamine 10 μg/kg min. Immediately after admission to the ICU, continuous hemodiafiltration (CHDF) was started without removal of water, because the echocardiographic examination revealed a relatively small left atrium and left ventricle, although his body weight (49.1 kg), IDVG (7.0 l, 163 ml/kg), and PV-ICG (2.7 l, 63 ml/kg) at that time did not support hypovolemia. Colloidal solution 500 ml was given to overcome hypotension.

However, atrial fibrillation associated with a ventricular rate of 120–150/min subsequently developed. Thus, we decided to start withdrawal of water at a rate of 100 ml/h and to give digoxin 0.5 mg to overcome atrial fibrillation associated with tachycardia, despite a decreased cardiac preload as judged by echocardiography. Thereafter, his cardiovascular state improved without any further fluid volume loading. On the second postoperative morning, his body weight decreased to 46.5 kg, even though IDVG (7.8 l, 181 ml/kg) and PV-ICG (2.8 l, 65 ml/kg) remained elevated. He was discharged from the ICU to the surgical ward on the sixth postoperative day without requiring infusions of vasoactive drugs and CHDF.

Comments

In retrospect, this patient had been overhydrated when admitted to the ICU. We believe that echocardiographic examination cannot consistently give accurate information of cardiac preload, even though authorities strongly recommend use of echocardiography as a measure of cardiac preload.

14. Current Cardiac Preload Assessment

Rational decision making for cardiovascular and fluid management in critically ill patients requires reliable assessment of cardiac preload and circulating blood volume (CBV). Ideally, the technology should be safe, noninvasive, accurate, reliable, continuous, and available without expensive equipment. However, no single monitoring tool currently meets all these requirements. A misinterpretation of cardiac preload or CBV when each inaccuracy of the measurement is not recognized could bring serious consequences in critically ill patients.

Cardiac Filling Pressures

Pulmonary artery wedge pressure (PAWP) and central venous pressure (CVP) are known as cardiac filling pressures. Although routine hemodynamic variables such as arterial pressure, cardiac filling pressure, and hematocrit have generally been used as guides for fluid management, none of them consistently indicates the status of either circulating blood volume (CBV) (Shippy et al. 1984; Brock et al. 2002), central blood volume (intrathoracic blood volume) (Lichtwarck-Aschoff et al. 1992; Boussat et al. 2002), or ventricular preload (Kumar et al. 2004).

Echocardiography

Echocardiography has become popular in the ICU for evaluation of cardiac preload as well as cardiac function. The left ventricular end-diastolic area (LVEDA) measured using transesophageal echocardiography has been used as a measure of cardiac preload. Alternatively, the characteristics of the Doppler flow-velocity waveform provide information on cardiac preload as well. The left ventricular ejection time (or flow time) corrected for heart rate provides an index of preload (Marik 1999). However, echocardiography cannot consistently be utilized, because an adequate view of cardiac chambers cannot be obtained, particularly after thoracic and/or upper abdominal surgical procedures such as the radical operation for esophageal carcinoma in which postoperative hemodynamic instability is frequently encountered.

Additionally, echocardiographic evaluation of fluid volume states is not consistently adequate because the cardiac chambers do not have a uniform shape among patients. Furthermore, preload is itself influenced not only by fluid volume states but also by changes in heart rate as observed during atrial pacing (Lancon et al. 1994). The shorter the filling interval, the smaller the cardiac filling volume. Considering these findings, echocardiography can identify an increase or decrease in cardiac preload but fails to identify small changes, as described in Chapter 13 (case 5), although echocardiographic assessment is generally recommended in critically ill patients. In fact, Bennett-Guerrero et al. (2002) found no relationship between left ventricular end-diastolic area and intravascular volume status in cardiac surgical patients.

Fluid Volume Challenge and Cardiac Filling Pressure Response

A fixed volume of colloid (e.g., 200 ml) is infused over 10–15 min, and the response in cardiac filling pressures is observed. The pattern of filling pressure response to a fluid challenge is not predictable simply from that pressure under different conditions. An elevated CVP or PAWP may decrease, increase, or remain the same in response to a fluid challenge (Grocott et al. 2005). This fluid volume challenge is generally more relevant than pressure monitoring alone but has the potential risk of producing overhydration associated with peripheral edema and/or congestive heart failure.

Systolic Pressure Variation

Systolic pressure variation (SPV) is fluctuation in systolic arterial blood pressure and has been shown to be related to stroke volume variation with positive pressure ventilation. SPV is defined as the difference between the maximal and minimal values of systolic arterial pressure recorded over a respiratory cycle. Normal SPV value is less than 10 mmHg (Parry-Jones and Pittman 2003). One may predict preload responsiveness because the greater the amplitude of ventilation-associated arterial pressure variation, the greater the patient's preload responsiveness (Gunn and Pinsky 2001). Although SPV has a potentially more accurate measure of preload responsiveness, cardiac surgical patients before cardiopulmonary bypass failed to demonstrate a relationship between SPV and subsequent response to a volume challenge (Bennett-Guerrero et al. 2002). Furthermore, this approach consistently requires mechanical ventilation with a constant tidal volume and a fixed respiratory rate and sinus rhythm (Parry-Jones and Pittman 2003). These requirements are found only in a limited number of ICU patients.

Intrathoracic Blood Volume

Measurement of intrathoracic blood volume (ITBV) using the single transpulmonary dilution technique is now used in several ICUs, particularly in Europe, as this technique is a more clinically relevant measure of cardiac preload than cardiac filling pressures. Considering the basic principle of this technique, however, mean transit time (MTT) of the indicator substance (e.g., cold saline) has a significant impact on determining ITBV as equivalent to cardiac output (CO) (as described in Chapter 11). Assuming that MTT is prolonged even if CO is low, the calculated ITBV would be normal or even increased. Subsequent hypovolemic hypotension after admission to the ICU has been frequently observed even in patients whose ITBV was normal or even increased at admission to the ICU after esophagectomy (Ishihara et al. 2005b). Presumably, this technique cannot consistently predict hypovolemic hypotension early after esophagectomy or is not consistently accurate in the presence of left ventricular dysfunction (as described in Chapter 10). Additionally, this approach requires an invasive procedure (placement of the femoral artery probe) in addition to routine arterial and central venous lines.

Right Ventricular End-Diastolic Volume

A thermodilution pulmonary artery catheter with a rapid response thermistor for continuous monitoring of CO, right ventricular ejection fraction (RVEF), and right ventricular end-diastolic volume (RVEDV) has become available in the operating room and in the ICU. RVEDV has been shown to be a better indicator of cardiac preload than cardiac filling pressures (Kincaid et al. 2001), and reported normal indexed RVEDV (RVEDVI) ranges from 90 to 140 ml/m^2 (Marik 1999).

The most important disadvantage of this method is that RVEDV is calculated based on RVEF and CO. The change in RVEF reflects the change in right ventricular (RV) function but does not mean the change in intrinsic RV contractility (Boldt et al. 1989). Gödje et al. (1998) reported a poor correlation between RVEDVI and stroke volume index (SVI) or cardiac index (CI), despite a good correlation between ITBVI and SVI or CI in cardiac surgical patients. Another limitation of this method is that it provides only averaged information but not real-time information regarding changes in RVEF and RV volume. Tricuspid regurgitation and rhythm disturbance reduce the accuracy of measured variables derived from this catheter (Kwak et al. 2004).

Indocyanine Green Pulse Dye Densitometry

CBV has been wrongly used as a measure of cardiac preload because CBV fails to decrease despite redistribution of fluid from the central to peripheral compartment, as described in Chapter 9. However, measurement of CBV is desirable for rational fluid management, which is currently based solely on cardiac filling pressures. A relatively noninvasive indocyanine green (ICG) dilution method for measuring CBV with pulse dye densitometry (ICG-PDD) has become clinically possible (Haruna et al. 1998; Iijima et al. 1998; He et al. 1998; Imai et al. 2000), although CBV does not consistently indicate cardiac preload. We checked the accuracy of this method in postcardiac surgical patients using calculated plasma volume from CBV-derived ICG-PDD and hematocrit (PV-PDD) (Ishihara et al. 2002).

Reviewing each dye dilution curve of ICG-PDD associated with the computed regression line revealed that 20 of these 47 recordings were judged as completely adequate because the curve and the line looked identical, 23 recordings were judged as adequate as they seemed close, and the remaining 4 recordings were judged as inadequate because they looked different (Fig. 14-1). Simultaneously recorded ICG-PDD-derived cardiac output (CO-PDD) was found to overestimate thermodilution CO (CO-TD) by an average of 0.5 ± 2.1 l/min. Using ICG-derived plasma volume (PV-ICG) derived by a conventional sampling method and CO-TD as references, the relationship of inaccuracy between PV-PDD and CO-PDD was examined. Over- or underestimation of PV-PDD correlated with those of CO-PDD ($r = 0.57$, $n = 46$, $P < 0.001$) (Fig. 14-2). Presumably, over- or underestimation of PV-PDD would occur simultaneously with those of CO-PDD.

The extremely high or low PV-PDD/IDVG ratios observed in this study cannot be clinically negligible compared with PV-ICG. Haruna et al. (1998) compared PDD-derived CBV by using a nostril probe with the conventional blood sampling method for ICG determination in 27 cardiac surgical patients. They found the difference of CBV in the two methods was −0.23 ± 0.37 l. Imai et al. (2000) reported blood volume measured both by ICG-PDD at a nostril and by ^{51}Cr-labeled red blood cells after cardiac surgery. The difference between the two blood volumes was 0.26 ± 0.49 l. Although they concluded

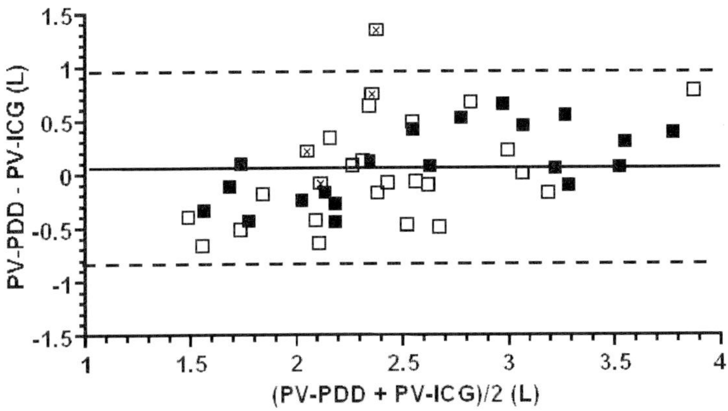

FIG. 14-1. Differences between PV-ICG and PV-PDD versus their mean values according to Bland and Altman's method associated with reviewed results of each ICG-PDD curve: completely adequate [■], adequate [□], or inadequate [⊠]. *PV-ICG*, conventional indocyanine green dilution-derived plasma volume requiring repeated blood sampling; *PV-PDD*, indocyanine green pulse dye densitometry-derived plasma volume. *Dashed lines* represent 95% confidence limits. (From Ishihara et al. (2002), p 785, fig. 2, with permission from Lippincott Williams & Wilkins)

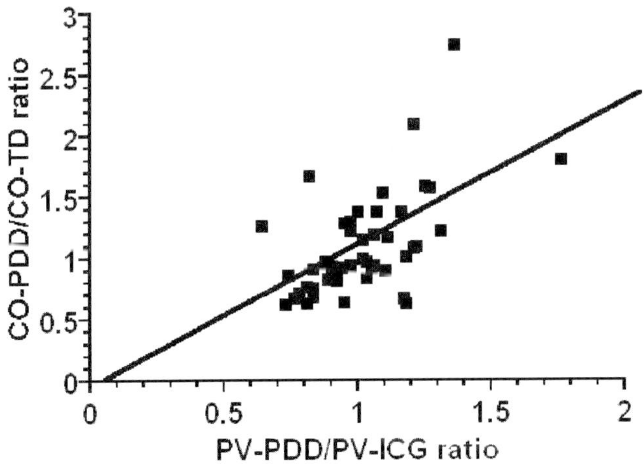

FIG. 14-2. Relationship of inaccuracy between PV-PDD and CO-PDD using PV-ICG and CO-TD as references. *PV-PDD*, pulse dye densitometry-derived plasma volume; *CO-PDD*, pulse dye densitometry-derived cardiac output; *PV-ICG*, conventional indocyanine green dilution-derived plasma volume requiring repeated blood sampling; *CO-TD*, continuous thermodilution cardiac output ($Y = 1.2X + 0.07$, $r = 0.57$, $n = 46$, $P < 0.001$). (From Ishihara et al. (2002), p 785, fig. 3, with permission from Lippincott Williams & Wilkins)

that ICG-PDD can measure blood volume with a small bias compared with the radioisotopic method, there was a similar bias as observed in this study (0.04 ± 0.44 l).

A considerable number of recordings were (13%) associated with a relatively low oxygen saturation at a nostril compared with the corresponding Pao_2 before ICG injection. An infusion of vasoactive drugs was also required on all but one occasion. Furthermore, subsequent hypovolemic hypotension requiring volume loading frequently developed within 2h after the first measurement. Considering these findings, poor peripheral circulation at a nostril is possible during data collection, leading to inaccurate estimation of absolute values of the blood ICG concentration, even though disappearance rate of ICG from blood using ICG-PDD was reported to be reliable in critical conditions (Sakka et al. 2000b). The inaccuracy is probably due to lack of high and stable oxygen saturation, adequate peripheral circulation, and/or unchanged probe position during data collection. Additionally, tissue factors that would affect the measurement of the dye concentration at each detection site may also play a role (Imai et al. 2000). Thus, these undesirable underlying conditions would limit the effectiveness and accuracy of the currently available ICG-PDD, and reviewing each ICG dilution curve alone does not consistently identify the inaccuracy. More sophisticated ICG-PDD is required to be used as a clinically relevant bedside monitor, even though the present ICG-PDD has been reported to be useful in the operating room (Haruna et al. 1998; He et al. 1998).

Inaccurate Fluid Volume Therapy

We believe that vasoactive agents are only required for patients who remain hemodynamically unstable or have evidence of tissue hypoxia even after adequate volume has been restored (Ishihara 2000a). Inadequate pharmacological support of circulation may follow instead of fluid administration or restriction when fluid volume status is not evaluated adequately. Consequently, reduced oxygen supply to several important organs such as kidneys and gastrointestinal tract can occur from reduced blood flow or increased interstitial edema, resulting in a significant increase in morbidity and mortality as well as length of hospital stay in critically ill patients (Sinclair et al. 1997; Gan et al. 2002; Venn et al. 2002). Optimization of stroke volume and other variables of oxygen delivery have been proposed in some randomized clinical trials to reduce complication and postoperative length of stay (Sinclair et al. 1997; Gan et al. 2002). The goal of volume challenge guided by stroke volume was to expand the intravascular volume and avoid hypovolemia without threatening a failing myocardium.

Assuming that fluid therapy is based solely on cardiac filling or intrathoracic blood volume status, or even based on stroke volume measurement, the following results would occur in the absence of reliable information of CBV status.

When cardiac preload is low in association with normal or even higher CBV, namely, central hypovolemia and peripheral blood pooling, additional further fluid resuscitation based on a low cardiac preload would yield excessive peripheral edema formation and subsequently pulmonary dysfunction and prolonged need for mechanical ventilation (Thorborg and Haupt 2000). In contrast, when cardiac preload is high, associated with normal or even low CBV because of increased sympathetic activity, restriction of fluid or administration of diuretics would produce a decrease in gut perfusion, resulting in intramucosal ischemia and acidosis (Wardrop et al. 1992).

Either of these sequelae would affect the outcome of critically ill patients (Wardrop et al. 1992; Sinclair et al. 1997). Therefore, we believe that assessment of these two blood volume states, namely, central and circulating blood volume states, is equally important for decision making in hemodynamic, fluid, and blood transfusion management.

IDVG and Future Investigation

We have proposed the initial distribution volume of glucose (IDVG) measurement, which is useful as a measure of the central extracellular fluid (ECF) volume even during hemodynamically unstable, even though IDVG cannot be used directly as a surrogate measure of cardiac preload. Our experience with more than 4000 IDVG determinations allows us to conclude that the central ECF volume status plays a role equally important as cardiac preload in maintaining stable hemodynamics, even though the former compared to the latter has been ignored in cardiovascular and fluid management. IDVG measurement can be simply, rapidly, and reliably performed in critically ill patients without the use of either a toxic indicator or expensive equipment. It requires only a small amount of glucose, arterial and central venous lines, and a conventional glucose analyzer in the ICU. Its repeated measurement is possible at 30-min intervals.

Considering inaccurate fluid management based on cardiac preload alone, however, simultaneous assessment of CBV or plasma volume in addition to

IDVG measurement would make fluid and/or blood transfusion therapy much more rational than at present. Furthermore, we believe noninvasive technology will also be available to accurately measure ICG and glucose in blood in the near future. These two fluid volumes would provide benefit in terms of point-of-care testing in critically ill patients. However, it remains unclear whether we should simply aim for normal central or circulating blood volume in critically ill patients, because optimal fluid volume status may vary with each individual patient as well as with the underlying pathology. This pathway is another subject that will need future investigation.

References

Akaike H (1985) A new look at the statistical model identification. IEEE Trans Autom Control AC-19:16–23

Avram MJ, Krejcie TC, Henthorn TK (1990) The relationship of age to the pharmacokinetics of early drug distribution: the concurrent disposition of thiopental and indocyanine green. Anesthesiology 72:403–411

Avram MJ, Kericie TC, Niemann CU, Enders-Klein C, Shanks CA, Henthorn TK (2000) Isoflurane alters the recirculatory pharmacokinetics of physiologic markers. Anesthesiology 92:1757–1768

Baluna R, Vitetta ES (1997) Vascular leak syndrome: a side effect of immunotherapy. Immunopharmacology 37:117–132

Bauer K, Versmold H, Prolss A, De Graaf SS, Meeuwsen Van Der Roest WP, Versmold H, Zijlstra WG (1990) Estimation of extracellular volume in preterm infants less than 1500 g, children, and adults by sucrose dilution. Pediatr Res 27:256–259

Bennet LZ, Sheiner LB (1985) Pharmacokinetics: the dynamics of drug absorption, disposition, and elimination. In: Goodman Gilman A, Foodman LS, Rall TW, Murad F (eds) The pharmacological basis of therapeutics. Macmillian, New York, pp 3–34

Bennett-Guerrero E, Kahn RA, Moskowitz DM, Falcucci O, Bodian CA (2002) Comparison of arterial systolic pressure variation with other clinical parameters to predict the response to fluid challenges during cardiac surgery. Mt Sinai J Med 69:96–100

Benya R, Quaintana J, Brundage B (1989) Adverse reactions to indocyanine green: a case report and a review of the literature. Catheter Cardiovasc Diagn 17:231–233

Biddle TL, Khanna PK, Yu PN, Hodges M, Shah PM (1973) Lung water in patients with acute myocardial infarction. Circulation 48:115–123

Bindels AJGH, van der Hoeven JG, Graafland AD, de Koning J, Meinders AE (2000) Relationships between volume and pressure measurements and stroke volume in critically ill patients. Crit Care 4:193–199

Boldt J, Kling D, Bormann BV, Scheld HH, Hempelmann G (1987) Influence of cardiac output on thermal-dye extravascular lung water (EVLW) in cardiac patients. Intensive Care Med 13:310–314

Boldt J, Kling D, Moosdorf P, Hempelmann G (1989) Influence of acute volume loading on right ventricular function after cardiopulmonary bypass. Crit Care Med 17:518–522

Boldt J (2000) Volume replacement in the surgical patient: does the type of solution make a difference? Br J Anaesth 84:783–793

Bone RC, Balk RA, Cerra FB, Dellinger RP, Fein AM, Knaus WA, Schein RM, Sibbald WJ (1992) Definitions for sepsis and organ failure and guidelines for the use of innovative therapies in sepsis: the ACCP/SCCM Consensus Conference Committee. American College of Chest Physicians/Society of Critical Care Medicine. Chest 101:1644–1655

Bonnet F, Richard C, Glaser P, Lafay M, Guesde R (1982) Changes in hepatic flow induced by continuous positive pressure ventilation in critically ill patients. Crit Care Med 10:703–705

Boussat S, Jacques B, Levy B, Laurent E, Gache A, Capellier G, Neidhardt A (2002) Intravascular volume monitoring and extravascular lung water in septic patients with pulmonary edema. Intensive Care Med 28:712–718

Brauer KI, Svensen C, Hahn RG, Traber LD, Prough DS (2002) Volume kinetic analysis of the distribution of 0.9% saline in conscious versus isoflurane-anesthetized sheep. Anesthesiology 96:442–449

Brigham KL, Bowers R, Haynes J (1979) Increased sheep lung vascular permeability caused by *Escherichia coli* endotoxin. Circ Res 45:292–297

Brock H, Gabriel C, Bibl D, Necek S (2002) Monitoring intravascular volumes for postoperative volume therapy. Eur J Anaesth 19:288–294

Buhre W, Bendyk K, Weyland A, Kazmaier S, Schmidt M, Mursch M, Sonntag H (1998) Assessment of intrathoracic blood volume. Thermo-dye dilution technique vs. single-thermodilution technique. Anaesthesist 47:51–53

Busse MW, Zisowsky S, Henschen S, Panning B, Piepenbrock S (1993) Plasma volume estimation using indocyanine green. Anaesthesia 48:41–43

Chinkes D, deMelo E, Zhang X-J (1995) Increased plasma glucose clearance in sepsis is due to increased exchange between plasma and interstitial fluid. Shock 4:356–360

Clancy TV, Norman K, Reynolds R, Covington D, Maxwell JG (1991) Cardiac output measurement in critical care patients: thoracic electrical bioimpedance versus thermodilution. J Trauma 31:1116–1121

Cobelli C, Bier DM, Ferrannini E (1990) Modeling glucose metabolism in man: theory and practice. Horm Metab Res 24(suppl):1–10

Cunningham VJ, Heath DF (1978) An interpretation of the intravenous glucose tolerance test in the light of recent findings on the kinetics of glucose and insulin in man. Clin Sci Mol Med 54:161–173

Da Luz PL, Weil MH, Liu VY, Shubin H (1974) Plasma volume prior to and following volume loading during shock complicating acute myocardial infarction. Circulation 49:98–105

Della Rocca G, Costa GM, Coccia C, Pompei L, Di Marco P, Pietropaoli P (2002) Preload index: pulmonary artery occlusion pressure versus intrathoracic blood volume monitoring during lung transplantation. Anesth Analg 95:835–843

Dembling RH (1987) Fluid replacement in burned patients. Surg Clin N Am 67:15–30

Diaz-Parejo P, Stahl N, Xu W, Reinstrup P, Ungerstedt U, Nordstrom CH (2003) Cerebral energy metabolism during transient hyperglycaemia in patients with severe brain trauma. Intensive Care Med 29:544–550

D'Orio V, Wahelen C, Naldi M, Fossion A, Junchmes J, Marcelle R (1989) Contribution of peripheral blood pooling to central hemodynamic disturbances during endotoxin insult in intact dogs. Crit Care Med 17:1314–1319

Dumont L, Lamoureux C, Lelorier J, Stanley P, Chartrand C (1982) Intravenous infusion of phentolamine: effects on cardiovascular dynamics and regional blood flow distribution in conscious dogs. J Cardiovasc Pharmacol 4:1055–1061

Ferrannini E, Smith JD, Cobelli C, Toffolo G, Pilo A, DeFronzo R (1985) Effect of insulin on the distribution and disposition of glucose in man. J Clin Invest 76:357–364

Fleck A, Raines G, Hawker F, Trotter J, Wallace PI, Ledingham IM, Calman KC (1985) Increased vascular permeability: a major cause of hypoalbuminaemia in disease and injury. Lancet 1:781–784

Fogh-Andersen N, Wimberley PD, Thode J, Siggard-Andersen O (1990) Direct reading glucose electrodes detect the molality of glucose in plasma and whole blood. Clin Chem Acta 189:33–38

Friedman Z, Berkenstadt H, Margalit N, Margalit N, Sega E, Perel A (2002) Cardiac output assessed by arterial thermodilution during exsanguination and fluid resuscitation: experimental validation against a reference technique. Eur J Anaesth 19:337–340

Gabbanelli V, Pntanetti S, Donati A, Montozzi A, Carbini C, Pelaia P (2004) Initial distribution volume of glucose as noninvasive indicator of cardiac preload: comparison with intrathoracic blood volume. Intensive Care Med 30:2067–2073

Gan TJ, Soppitt A, Maroof M, el-Moalem H, Robertson KM, Moretti E, Dwane P, Glass PS (2002) Goal-directed intraoperative fluid administration reduces length of hospital stay after major surgery. Anesthesiology 97:820–826

Genoni M, Pelosi P, Romand JA, Pedoto A, Moccetti T, Malacrida R (1998) Determination of cardiac output during mechanical ventilation by electrical bioimpedance or thermodilution in patients with acute lung injury: effects of positive end-expiratory pressure. Crit Care Med 26:1441–1445

Ghoneim M, Pearson K (1990) Pharmacokinetics of drugs administered intravenously. In: Scurr C, Feldman S, Soni N (eds) Scientific foundations of anaesthesia, 4th edn. Year Book Medical, Chicago, pp 559–571

Giddings AE, Mangnall D, Rowlands BJ, Clark RG (1977) Plasma insulin and surgery. I. Early changes due to operation in the insulin response to glucose. Ann Surg 186:681–686

Gödje O, Peyerl M, Seebauer T, Lamm P, Mair H, Reinhart B (1998) Central venous pressure, pulmonary capillary wedge pressure and intrathoracic blood volumes as preload indicators in cardiac surgery patients. Eur J Cardiothorac Surg 13:533–540

Gödje O, Thiel C, Lamm P, Reichenspurner H, Schmitz C, Schutz A, Reichart B (1999) Less invasive, continuous hemodynamic monitoring during minimally invasive coronary surgery. Ann Thorac Surg 68:1532–1536

Gödje O, Seebauer T, Peyerl M, Pfeiffer UJ, Reichart B (2000) Hemodynamic monitoring by double-indicator dilution technique in patients after orthotopic heart transplantation. Chest 118:775–781

Gold MS (1992) Perioperative fluid management. Crit Care Clin 8:409–421

Grocott MPW, Mythen MG, Gan TJ (2005) Perioperative fluid management and clinical outcome in adults. Anesth Analg 100:1093–1106

Gunn SR, Pinsky MR (2001) Implications of arterial pressure variation in patients in the intensive care unit. Curr Opin Crit Care 7:212–217

Guyton AC, Hall JE (2000a) Textbook of medical physiology, 10th edn. Saunders, Philadelphia, pp 162–183

Guyton AC, Hall JE (2000b) Textbook of medical physiology, 10th edn. Saunders, Philadelphia, pp 264–278

Hahn RG (1996) Glucose kinetics in haemorrhagic shock (correspondence). Eur J Anaesth 13:213

Hahn RG (2005) Blood glucose increments as a measure of body physiology. Crit Care 9:155–157

Haller M, Akbulut C, Brechtelsbauer AH, Fett W, Briegel J, Finsterer U, Peter K (1993) Determination of plasma volume with indocyanine green in man. Life Sci 53:1597–1604

Haruna M, Kumon K, Yahagi N, Watanabe Y, Ishida Y, Kobayashi N, Aoyagi T (1998) Blood volume measurement at the bedside using ICG pulse spectrophotometry. Anesthesiology 89:1322–1328

Harvey M, Voss L, Sleigh J (2003) Preload response in patients after cardiac surgery: a comparison of systolic pressure and systolic area variability and initial distribution volume of glucose. Crit Care Resusc 5:171–176

Hashimoto H, Ishihara H (1997) PFK and immune function. In: Matsuki A, Ishihara H (eds) Clinical application of total intravenous anesthesia (in Japanese). Kokuseidoh, Tokyo, pp 83–92

He YL, Tanigami H, Ueyama H, Mashimo T, Yoshiya I (1998) Measurement of blood volume using indocyanine green measured with pulse-spectrophotometry: its reproducibility and reliability. Crit Care Med 26:1446–1451

Hedenstierna G (1992) What value does the recording of intrathoracic blood volume have in clinical practice? Intensive Care Med 18:137–138

Hemstad JR, Spiess BD, Marchioro TL, Raghu G (1994) Pulmonary artery and non-invasive hemodynamics during lung lavage in primary alveolar proteinosis. Chest 105:1605–1608

Henschen S, Busse MW, Zisowsky S, Panning B (1993) Determination of plasma volume and total blood volume using indocyanine green: a short review. J Med 24:10–27

Henthorn TK, Avram MJ, Kejcie TC (1989) Intravascular mixing and drug distribution: the concurrent disposition of thiopental and indocyanine green. Clin Pharmacol Ther 45:56–65

Hirota K, Ishihara H, Tsubo T, Matsuki A (1999) Estimation of the initial distribution volume of glucose by an incremental plasma glucose level at 3 minutes after i.v. glucose in humans. Br J Clin Pharmacol 47:361–364

Hoeft A, Schorn B, Weyland A, Scholz M, Buhre W, Stepanek E (1994) Bedside assessment of intravascular volume status in patients undergoing coronary bypass surgery. Anesthesiology 81:76–86

Hoffman BB, Leftkowitz RJ (1996) Catecholamines, sympathomimetic drugs, and adrenergic receptor antagonists. In: Hardann JG (ed) Goodman & Gilman's: the pharmacological basis of therapeutics, 9th edn. McGraw-Hill, New York, pp 199–248

Hull CJ (1991) Pharmacokinetics for anaesthesia. Butterworth-Heinemann, Oxford, pp 3–16

Hwang SW (1975) Plasma and hepatic binding of indocyanine green in guinea pigs of different ages. Am J Physiol 228:718–724

Iijima T, Iwao Y, Sankawa H (1998) Circulating blood volume measured by pulse dye-densitometry: comparison with ^{131}I-RISA analysis. Anesthesiology 89:1329–1335

Imai T, Mitaka C, Koike A, Ohki S, Isa Y, Kunimoto F (2000) Accuracy and repeatability of blood volume measurement by pulse dye densitometry compared to the conventional method using ^{51}Cr-labeled red blood cells. Intensive Care Med 26:1343–1349

Imu A, Charlson RW (1993) Fluid resuscitation in circulatory shock. Crit Care Clin 9:313–333

Insel PA, Liljenquist JE, Tobin JD, Sherwin RS, Watkins P, Andres R, Berman M (1975) Insulin control of glucose metabolism in man. J Clin Invest 55:1057–1066

Ishibe Y, Suekane K (1984) Method of measuring lung water and a few problems (in Japanese). Jpn J Intensive Care Med 8:177–187

Ishigami Y, Masuzawa M, Miyoshi E, Kato M, Tamura K, Kanda M, Awazu K, Taniguchi K, Kurita M, Hayashi N, Kawano S, Fusamoto H, Kamada T (1993) Clinical applications of ICG finger monitor in patients with liver disease. J Hepatol 19:232–240

Ishihara H, Kallus FT, Giesecke AH (1981) Intravenous glucose tolerance test during anaesthesia in dogs: insulin response and glucose clearance. Can Anaesth Soc J 28:381–386

Ishihara H, Yao M, Amano N, Shirasaki S, Kudo T, Matsuki A, Oyama T (1985) Metabolic and endocrine response to anesthesia and surgery during trimetaphan infusion in man (in Japanese). Masui 34:626–631

Ishihara H, Tanioka F, Matsuki A, Katagai H, Sakai T, Oyama T (1986a) Changes in postoperative glucose space in ICU (in Japanese). J Water Electrolyte Metab 6:75–79

Ishihara H, Tanioka F, Katagai H, Sakai T, Kudo T, Matsuki A, Oyama T (1986b) Effects of anesthesia and surgery on glucose space in man (in Japanese). Masui 35:1057–1062

Ishihara H, Shimodate Y, Koh H, Isozaki K, Tsubo T, Matsuki A (1993) The initial distribution volume of glucose and cardiac output in the critically ill. Can J Anaesth 40:28–31

Ishihara H, Takamura K, Koh H, Iwakawa T, Tsubo T, Matsuki A (1996a) Does the initial distribution volume of glucose reflect the central extracellular fluid volume status in critically ill patients? Infusionsther Transfusionsmed 23:196–201

Ishihara H, Matsuno S, Taguchi S, Araki I, Tsubo T, Matsuki A (1996b) Evaluation of fluid volume status with a glucose challenge test in a patient with acute adrenal insufficiency. J Anesth 10:69–71

Ishihara H (1996c) Glucose kinetics in haemorrhagic shock (in reply). Eur J Anaesth 13:213–214

Ishihara H, Ohkawa H, Iwakawa T, Takamura K, Tsubo T, Matsuki A (1997) Possible overestimation of plasma volume determined by the indocyanine dilution method in the presence of protein leak from capillary beds: a discussion of two clinical cases. Infusionsther Transfusionsmed 24:10–13

Ishihara H, Otomo N, Suzuki A, Takamura K, Tsubo T, Matsuki A (1998a) Detection of capillary protein leakage by glucose and indocyanine green dilutions during the early post-burn period. Burns 24:525–531

Ishihara H, Suzuki A, Takamura K, Yatsu Y, Kimura N, Otomo N, Tsubo T, Matsuki A (1998b) Does the initial distribution volume of glucose reflect the shift of the central extracellular fluid volume after major surgical procedures? (in Japanese). J Jpn Intensive Care Med 5:203–210

Ishihara H, Iwakawa T, Hasegawa Y, Muraoka M, Tsubo T, Matsuki A (1999) Does indocyanine green accurately measure plasma volume independently of its disappearance rate from plasma in critically ill patients? Intensive Care Med 25:1252–1258

Ishihara H (2000a) Measurement of blood volume in the ICU (review). Int J Intensive Care 7:142–150

Ishihara H (2000b) Hemodynamic assessment and monitoring. In: Matsuki A, Ishihara H (eds) Patients management during early after surgery, 2nd edn (In Japanese). Kokuseidoh, Tokyo, pp 275–279

Ishihara H, Suzuki A, Okawa H, Sakai I, Tsubo T, Matsuki A (2000c) The initial distribution volume of glucose rather than indocyanine green derived plasma volume is correlated with cardiac output following major surgery. Intensive Care Med 26:1441–1448

Ishihara H, Matsui A, Muraoka M, Tanabe T, Tsubo T, Matsuki A (2000d) Detection of capillary leakage by the indocyanine green and glucose dilutions in septic patients. Crit Care Med 28:620–626

Ishihara H, Suzuki A, Okawa H, Ebina T, Tsubo T, Matsuki A (2001) Comparison of the initial distribution volume of glucose and plasma volume in thoracic fluid-accumulated patients. Crit Care Med 29:1532–1538

Ishihara H, Okawa H, Iwakawa T, Umegaki N, Tsubo T, Matuski A (2002) Does indocyanine green accurately measure plasma volume early after cardiac surgery? Anesth Analg 94:781–786

Ishihara H, Nakamura H, Okawa H, Takase H, Tsubo T, Hirota K (2005a) Initial distribution volume of glucose can be approximated using a conventional glucose analyzer in the intensive care unit. Crit Care 9:R144–R149

Ishihara H, Nakamura H, Okawa H, Yatsu Y, Tsubo T, Hirota K (2005b) Comparison of initial distribution volume of glucose and intrathoracic blood volume during hemodynamically unstable states early after esophagectomy. Chest 128:1713–1719

Ishihara H (2006) Initial distribution volume of glucose early after cardiac surgery (letter to the editor). Anesth Analg 102:1904

Iwakawa T, Ishihara H, Takamura K, Sakai I, Suzuki A (1998) Measurements of extracellular fluid volume in highly perfused organs and lung water in hypo- and hypervolaemic dogs. Eur J Anaesth 15:414–421

Jones JG, Wardrop CAJ (2000) Measurement of blood volume in surgical and intensive care practice. Br J Anaesth 84:226–235

Junghans T, Bohm B, Hasse O, Fritzmann J, Zuckermann-Becker H (2002) Conventional monitoring and intravascular volume measurement can lead to different therapy after upper gastrointestinal tract surgery. Intensive Care Med 28:1273–1275

Karcher RE, Ingram RL, Kiechle FL, Sykes E (1993) Comparison of the HomoCue berta-glucose photometer and reflotron for open heart surgery. Am J Clin Pathol 100:130–134

Keith NM, Power MH (1937) The urinary excretion of sucrose and its distribution in the blood after intravenous injection into normal men. Am J Physiol 120:203–210

Kholoussy AM, Pollack D, Matsumoto T (1984) Prognostic significance of indocyanine green clearance in critically ill surgical patients. Crit Care Med 12:115–116

Kincaid EH, Meredith JW, Chang MC (2001) Determining optimal cardiac preload during resuscitation using measurements of ventricular compliance. J Trauma 50:665–659

Knaus WA, Draper EA, Wagner DP, Zimmerman JE (1985) APACHE 2: a severity of disease classification system. Crit Care Med 13:818–828

Koh H, Ishihara H, Miyahara A, Matsuki A (1995) Does the initial distribution volume of glucose reflect plasma volume after haemorrhage in dogs? Can J Anaesth 42:163–167

Kumar A, Anel R, Bunnell E, Habet K, Zanotti S, Marshall S, Neumann A, Ali A, Cheang M, Kavinsky C, Parrillo JE (2004) Pulmonary artery occlusion pressure and central venous pressure fail to predict ventricular filling volume, cardiac performance, or the response to volume infusion in normal subjects. Crit Care Med 32:691–699

Kurahashi K, Maruta H, Usuda Y, Ohtsuka M (1997) Influence of blood sample oxygen tension on blood glucose concentration measured using an enzyme-electrode method. Crit Care Med 25:231–235

Kuwa K, Nakayama T, Hoshino T, Tominaga M (2001) Relationships of glucose concentrations in capillary whole blood, venous whole blood and venous plasma. Clin Chem Acta 307:187–192

Kwak YL, Oh YJ, Jung SM, Yoo KJ, Lee JH, Hong YW (2004) Change in right ventricular function during off-pump coronary artery bypass graft surgery. Eur J Cardiothorac Surg 25:572–577

Lancon JP, Pillet M, Gabrielle F, Fayolle JL, Tatou E (1994) Effects of atrial pacing on right ventricular contractility after coronary artery surgery. J Cardiothorac Vasc Anesth 8:536–540

Levin VA, Fenstermacher JD, Patlak CS (1970) Sucrose and inulin space measurements of cerebral cortex in four mammalian species. Am J Physiol 219:1528–1533

Lichtwarck-Aschoff M, Zeravik J, Pfeiffer UJ (1992) Intrathoracic blood volume accurately reflects circulatory volume status in critically ill patients with mechanical ventilation. Intensive Care Med 18:142–147

Loo JCK, Riegelman S (1970) Assessment of pharmacokinetic constant from postinfusion blood curves obtained after IV infusion. J Pharm Sci 59:53–55

Marik PE (1999) Pulmonary artery catheterization and esophageal Doppler monitoring in the ICU. Chest 116:1085–1091

Marino PL (1997) The ICU book, 2nd edn. Williams & Wilkins, Philadelphia. pp 691–708

Maser RE, Butler MA, Decherney GS (1994) Use of arterial blood with bedside glucose reflectance meters in an intensive care unit: are they accurate? Crit Care Med 22:595–599

Matsui A, Ishihara H, Suzuki A, Hashiba E, Fukushi T, Matsuki A (2000) Glucose dilution can detect fluid redistribution following phentolamine infusion in dogs. Intensive Care Med 26:1131–1138

Maynard ND, Bihari DJ, Dalton RN, Beale R, Smithies MN, Mason RC (1997) Liver function and splanchnic ischemia in critically ill patients. Chest 111:180–187

McKee PA, Castelli WP, McNamara PA, Kannel WB (1971) The natural history of congestive heart failure: the Framingham study. N Engl J Med 285:1441–1445

Mi W-D, Ishihara H, Sakai T, Matsuki A (2003) Possible overestimation of indocyanine green-derived plasma volume early after induction of anesthesia with propofol/fentanyl. Anesth Analg 97:1421–1427

Miyahara A, Ohkawa H, Ishihara H, Matsuki A (1995) Changes in the initial distribution volume of glucose and plasma volume following volume challenge in dogs. Infusionsther Transfusionsmed 22:274–279

Moore FA, Haenel JB, Moore EE (1991) Alternatives to Swan–Ganz cardiac output monitoring. Surg Clin N Am 71:699–721

Mulrow PJ, Oestrich HM, Swan RC (1956) Measurement of extracellular fluid volume of nephrectomized dogs with mannitol, sucrose, thiosulfate and radiosulfate. Am J Physiol 185:179–184

Mundigler G, Heinze G, Zehetgruber M, Gabriel H, Siostrzonek P (2000) Limitations of the transpulmonary indicator dilution method for assessment of preload changes in critically ill patients with reduced left ventricular function. Crit Care Med 28:2231–2237

Nakamura H, Ishihara H, Okawa H, Yatsu Y, Tsubo T, Matsuki A (2005) Initial distribution volume of glucose is correlated with intrathoracic blood volume in hypovolemia and following volume loading in dogs. Eur J Anaesth 22:202–208

Nakanishi K, Takeda S, Terajima K, Takano T, Ogawa R (2000) Myocardial dysfunction associated with proinflammatory cytokines after esophageal resection. Anesth Analg 91:270–275

Neumann P (1999) Extravascular lung water and intrathoracic blood volume: double versus single indicator dilution technique. Intensive Care Med 25:216–219

Okumura S, Takeda A, Miyamoto T, Hagio M, Fujinaga T (1995) Transmigration of fluid rapidly infused into dogs with renal blood vessel ligation and increased pulmonary capillary permeability. J Vet Med Sci 57:213–218

Orth VH, Rehm M, Thiel M, Kreimeier U, Haller M, Brechtelsbauer H, Finsterer U (1998) First clinical implications of perioperative red cell volume measurement with a nonradioactive marker (sodium fluorescein). Anesth Analg 87:1234–1238

Parry-Jones AJD, Pittman JAL (2003) Arterial pressure and stroke volume variability as measurements for cardiovascular optimisation. Int J Intensive Care 10:67–72

Passmore JM (1985) Adrenal cortex. In: Geehoed GS, Chenow B (eds) Endocrine aspects of acute illness. Churchill Livingstone, New York, pp 97–134

Pearson TC, Guthrie DL, Simpson J, Chinn S, Barosi G, Ferrant A, Lewis SM, Najean Y (1995) Interpretation of measured red cell mass and plasma volume in adults: Expert Panel on Radionuclides of the International Council for Standardization in Haematology. Br J Haematol 89:748–756

Pomerantz M, Delgado F, Eiseman B (1970) Clinical evaluation of transthoracic electrical impedance as a guide to intrathoracic fluid volumes. Ann Surg 171:686–690

Preisman S, Pfeiffer U, Lieberman N, Perel A (1997) New monitors of intravascular volume: a comparison of arterial pressure waveform analysis and the intrathoracic blood volume. Intensive Care Med 23:651–657

Pruitt BA Jr (1978) Advances in fluid therapy and early care of the burned patient. World J Surg 2:139–150

Putensen C, Waibel U, Koller W, Putensen-Himmer G, Hormann C (1992) Assessment of changes in lung microvascular permeability in posttraumatic acute lung failure after direct and indirect injuries to lungs. Anesth Analg 74:793–799

Raisz LG, Young MK, Stinson IT (1953) Comparison of the volumes of distribution of inulin, sucrose and thiosulfate in normal and nephrectomized dogs. Am J Physiol 174:72–78

Rauch H, Müller M, Fleischer H, Bauer H, Martin E, Bottiger BW (2002) Pulse contour analysis versus thermodilution in cardiac surgical patients. Acta Anaesthesiol Scand 46:424–429

Ray JG, Hamielec C, Mastracci T (2001) Pilot study of the accuracy of bedside glucometry in the intensive care unit. Crit Care Med 29:2205–2207

Regittnig W, Trajanoski Z, Leis HJ, Ellmerer M, Wutte A, Sendlhofer G, Schaupp L, Brunner GA, Wach P, Pieber TR (1999) Plasma and interstitial glucose dynamics after intravenous glucose injection. Diabetes 48:1070–1081

Rehm M, Haller M, Brechtelsbauer C, Akbulut C, Finsterer U (1998) Extra protein loss not caused by surgical bleeding in patients with ovarian cancer. Acta Anaesthesiol Scand 42:39–46

Rehm M, Haller M, Orth V, Kreimeier U, Jacob M, Dressel H, Mayer S, Brechtelsbauer H, Finsterer U (2001) Changes in blood volume and hematocrit during acute preoperative volume loading with 5% albumin or 6% hetastarch solutions in patients before radical hysterectomy. Anesthesiology 95:849–856

Roos A, Westendorp RJ, Frolich M, Meinders AE (1993) Weight changes in critically ill patients evaluated by fluid balances and impedance measurements. Crit Care Med 21:871–877

Rose BO, Ishihara H, Okawa B, Panning B, Piepenbrock S, Matsuki A (2004) Repeatability of measurements of the initial distribution volume of glucose in haemodynamically stable patients. J Clin Pharm Ther 29:317–323
Rosenqvist U, Licko V, Karam JH (1976) Evaluation of a 'true' fractional removal rate of glucose in man by bolus and simulated-ramp increase of glucose. Diabetes 25:580–585
Sageman WS (1999) Reliability and precision of a new thoracic electrical bioimpedance monitor in a lower body negative pressure model. Crit Care Med 27: 1986–1990
Sakai I, Ishihara H, Iwakawa T, Suzuki A, Matsuki A (1998) Ratio of indocyanine green and glucose dilutions detects capillary protein leakage following endotoxin injection in dogs. Br J Anaesth 81:193–197
Sakka SG, Rühl CC, Pfeiffer UJ, Beale R, McLuckie A, Reinhart K, Meier-Hellmann A (2000a) Assessment of cardiac preload and extravascular lung water by single transpulmonary thermodilution. Intensive Care Med 26:180–187
Sakka SG, Reinhart K, Meier-Hellmann A (2000b) Comparison of invasive and noninvasive measurements of indocyanine green plasma disappearance rate in critically ill patients with mechanical ventilation and stable hemodynamics. Intensive Care Med 26:1553–1556
Savolainen K, Vitala A, Puhakainen E, Väisänen M (1990) Problems with the use of whole blood as a sample material in novel direct glucose analysers. Scand J Clin Lab Invest 50:221–223
Schroder T, Rosoler U, Ferichs I, Hahn G, Ennker J, Hellige G (1999) Errors of the back-extrapolation method in determination of the blood volume. Phys Med Biol 44:121–130
Schuster DP, Calandrino FS (1991) Single versus double indicator dilution measurements of extravascular lung water. Crit Care Med 19:84–88
Sekimoto M, Fukui M, Fujita K (1997) Plasma volume estimation using indocyanine green with biexponential regression analysis of the decay curves. Anaesthesia 52:1166–1172
Seltzer HS, Allen EW, Herron AL Jr, Brennan MT (1967) Insulin secretion in response to glycemic stimulus: relation of delayed initial release to carbohydrate intolerance in mild diabetes mellitus. J Clin Invest 46:323–335
Shimodate Y, Ishihara H, Matsuki A (1994) The initial distribution volume of glucose and cardiac output after haemorrhage in dogs. Can J Anaesth 41:257–260
Shimodate Y, Koh H, Ishihara H, Matsuki A (1995) Comparison of glucose and sucrose as an indicator for dilution volumetry in haemorrhagic shock. Eur J Anaesth 12:397–401
Shippy CR, Appel PL, Shoemaker WL (1984) Reliability of clinical monitoring to assess blood volume in critically ill patients. Crit Care Med 12:107–112
Sinclair S, James, Singer M (1997) Intraoperative intravascular volume optimisation and length of hospital stay after repair of proximal femoral fracture: randomised controlled trial. Br Med J 315:909–912
Steil GM, Richey J, Kim JK, Wi JK, Rebrin K, Bergman RN, Youn JH (1996) Extracellular glucose distribution is not altered by insulin: analysis of plasma and interstitial L-glucose kinetics. Am J Physiol 271:E855–E864
Suzuki A, Ishihara H, Hashiba E, Matsui A, Matsuki A (1999) Detection of histamine-induced capillary protein leakage and hypovolaemia by determination of indocyanine green and glucose dilution method in dogs. Intensive Care Med 25:304–310

Suzuki A, Ishihara H, Okawa H, Tsubo T, Matsuki A (2001) Can initial distribution volume of glucose predict hypovolemic hypotension after radical surgery for esophageal cancer? Anesth Analg 92:1146–1151

Takamura K, Iwakawa T, Sakai I, Muraoka M, Ishihara H, Matsuki A (1997) Comparison of the initial distribution volume of glucose and sucrose in volume-challenged dogs. Infusionsther Transfusionsmed 24:144–150

Thorborg P, Haupt MT (2000) Is it time to use blood volume measurements as a clinical tool? Crit Care Med 28:883–884

Tschaikowsky K, Meisner M, Durst R, Rugheimer E (1997) Blood volume determination using hydroxyethyl starch: a rapid and simple intravenous injection method. Crit Care Med 25:599–606

Valeri CR, Cooper AG, Pivacek LE (1973) Limitations of measuring blood volume with iodinated ^{125}I serum albumin. Arch Intern Med 132:534–538

Van De Water JM, Mount BE, Barela JR, Schuster R, Leacock FS (1973) Monitoring the chest with impedance. Chest 64:597–603

van Tulder L, Michaeli B, Chioléro R, Berger MM, Revelly JP (2005) An evaluation of the initial distribution volume of glucose to assess plasma volume during a fluid challenge. Anesth Analg 101:1089–1093

Venn R, Steele A, Richardson P, Poloniecki J, Grounds M, Newman P (2002) Randomized controlled trial to investigate influence of the fluid challenge on duration of hospital stay and perioperative morbidity in patients with hip fractures. Br J Anaesth 88:65–71

Vicini P, Caumo A, Cobelli C (1997) The hot IVGTT two-compartment minimal model: indexes of glucose effectiveness and insulin sensitivity. Am J Physiol 273: E1024–E1032

Wang HH, Liu LM, Katz RL (1977) A comparison of the cardiovascular effects of sodium nitroprusside and trimetaphan. Anesthesiology 46:40–48

Wang P, Zhang FB, Stephan MT, Mian Z, Irshad HC (1993) Alterations in circulating blood volume during polymicro sepsis. Circ Shock 40:92–98

Wardrop CAJ, Holland BM, Jacobs S, Jones JG (1992) Optimization of the blood for oxygen transport and tissue perfusion in critical care. Postgrad Med J 68(suppl 2): S2–S6

White HL, Rolf D (1958) Comparison of various procedures for determining sucrose and inulin space in the dog. J Clin Invest 37:8–19

Wick AN, Drury DR, Mackay EM (1950) Glucose space of the body. Am J Physiol 163:224–228

Wilmore DW, Mason AD Jr, Pruitt BA Jr (1976) Impaired glucose flow in burned patients with gram negative sepsis. Surg Gynecol Obstet 143:720–724

Wolfe RR, Elahi D, Spitzer JJ (1977) Glucose and lactate kinetics after endotoxin administration in dogs. Am J Physiol 232:E180–E185

Wolfe RR, Allsop JR, Burke JF (1978) Fallibility of the intravenous glucose tolerance test as a measure of endogenous glucose turnover. Metabolism 27:217–226

Yamaoka K, Tanigawara Y, Nakagawa T, Uno T (1981) A pharmacokinetic analysis program (MULTI) for microcomputers. J Pharm Dyn 4:879–885

Yamaoka K, Nakagawa T, Tanaka H, Yasuhara M, Okumura K, Hori R (1985) A nonlinear multiple regression program, MULTI 2 (Bayes), based on Bayesian algorithm for microcomputers. J Pharm Dyn 8:246–256

Youn JH, Kim JK, Steil GM (1995) Assessment of extracellular glucose distribution and glucose transport activity in conscious rats. Am J Physiol 268:E712–E721

Zarowitz BJ, Matthie JR (1999) Bioimpedance and the estimation of net fluid balance in critical care patients: problems and possibilities. Crit Care Med 27:1655–1657

Zöllner C, Goetz AE, Weis M, Mörstedt K, Pichler B, Lamm P, Kelger E, Haller M (2001) Continuous cardiac output measurements do not agree with conventional bolus thermodilution cardiac output determination. Can J Anesth 48:1143–1147

Zweens J, Frankena H (1980) Sucrose as an indicator for the measurement of the extracellular fluid volume in man. Proceedings of the 21st Dutch Federation Meeting, Nijmengen, the Netherlands

Subject Index